Pocket Handbook

of

Chinese Herbal

Prescriptions

350 Classic Formulas

By Zong Lan Xu

Published by

WACLION International Inc.

P. O. Box   163205

Miami, FL 33116-3205 USA

First Edition August 2001

Copyright © 2001 by Zong Lan Xu
Printed in the United States of America

Library of Congress Card number 00-140025

ISBN 0-9679935-1-2

Warning-Disclaimer

This book was designed to provide information as a professional reference only, not as a medical manual. A thorough knowledge of Chinese Medicine is required for purposes of treatment. Self diagnosis and medication is strongly discouraged. Practice of Chinese Medicine without license is against law.

The information presented in this book is given in good faith, however, there may be mistakes in typing, contents, and translating. Therefore, the author and publisher shall have neither liability nor responsibility to any treatment given with respect to any loss or damage caused, directly or indirectly by the information contained in this book.

Note From the Publisher

The author has made every effort to ensure this book accurate and user-friendly. However, your suggestions for improvement of future editions are appreciated. Please contact the publisher with your comments.

ii

Table of Contents

About The Author

Zong Lan Xu, is a doctor of Traditional Chinese Medicine from China. She was graduated from Shandong University of Traditional Chinese Medicine in 1982. She has been an educator and practitioner of Chinese medicine since then.

Dr.Xu has taught and lectured in different Oriental Medicine Institutes in China, United States, and Canada. She has published articles, papers, and books on Chinese Medicine in China and the United States. She was also part of an elite team that developed and propelled the National Certification Examination on Chinese Herbology and Acupuncture in the United States.

Dr.Xu is a faculty member of Southeast Institute of Oriental Medicine since 1991, and has a private practice in South Miami, Florida.

Acknowledgments

I would like to express my sincere thanks to all my teachers from Shandong University of Traditional Chinese Medicine, who have enabled me to write this book.

My deepest thanks to my dear friends, fellow classmates, Dr. Bing Ouyang, and Dr. Xinmin Gao who have given me some valuable suggestions and information for writing this book.

I am grateful to all my students who have encouraged me to publish this book.

To my lovely daughter, Linda, who helped me with typing and preparing documents, a special thank you.

My sincere appreciation to Margaret Sims for her help with technical editing, book design and typography; and Sherril Gold who designed the cover with her impressive artistic work.

A special thanks goes to Zyad Mohammed for his help in gathering marketing information on this project.

Introduction

This unique pocket handbook contains 350 classic Chinese herbal formulas. They are in alphabetical order by Chinese pinyin name. The information includes: Chinese name (both Chinese characters and pinyin); literally translated English name and alternate English name (if applicable); pertaining category; composed ingredients with recommended dosage; preparation; functions; indications; cautions; modern application; and comments. All information is based on textbooks used for national certification examination.

In order to understand the formulas correctly, the users must read the "Using the Guide" before studying this book.

Prior to all the individual formulas, there is a table of Chinese herbal formulas by functional categories with key pathological changes of each formula. The users can easily differentiate each formula from others in the same category and use them properly.

At the end, there are tables of clinical application of the formulas by differentiation according to Zang-fu organs, six stages, four levels, and triple burners. These will help users choose the best formula based on Traditional Chinese Medicine diagnosis for the patient.

This book is extremely handy and convenient for students, teachers, and practitioners using as a concise and quick reference. It will be also a good source for anyone who is looking for the information on classic Chinese herbal remedies.

Using the Guide

1. Symbols:

   ** Major and commonly used formulas

2. Dosage of ingredients

   1) The listed dosage of each ingredient in the formula is adult dosage based on textbooks and clinical experience. The dosage should be properly decreased in children.

   2) Most of listed dosages are for making decoction, while some are for making pills or powder, etc.

   3) Each decoction should be consumed within one day; the use of prepared forms (pill, tablet, powder, granular, capsule, extract, etc.) should follow the direction of each product from different manufacturers.

3. Modern application:

   The listed bio-medically defined disorders for each formula must have appropriate presentations (symptoms and signs) that match the traditional indications of the formula. The diagnosis of patient (based on Traditional Chinese Medicine) must conform to the treatment strategies of the formula. This methodology is called "Bian Zheng Lun Zhi", translated as "basing treatment on differentiation". According to this principle, one formula can be used for different diseases; and same disease can be treated with different formulas. These are called "Yi Bing Tong Zhi", "Tong Bing Yi Zhi" in Chinese Medicine.

4. Clinical application

Under each pattern, there are several formulas listed. Choose the best one or best combination for the patient based on the specialty of each formula and the constitution of each individual patient.

5. Special precaution

To avoid mercury poisoning, any formula that contains Zhu Sha (Cinnabar) should not be used long term.

Chinese Herbal Formulas by Functional Categories

Category	Formula Name	Key Pathological Changes
Pungent Warm Exterior Relieving 辛 温 解 表	***Ma Huang Tang* **** (Ephedra Decoction)	Wind-cold invasion with exterior excess
	San Ao Tang (Three Stubborn Decoction)	Mild wind-cold invasion affecting the lungs
	Da Qing Long Tang (Major Bluegreen Dragon Decoction)	Exterior wind-cold with interior heat
	Hua Gai San (Canopy Powder)	Wind-cold affecting the lungs with retention of phlegm
	Gui Zhi Tang* * (Cinnamon Twig Decoction)	Wind-cold invasion with exterior deficiency
	Ge Gen Tang (Pueraria Decoction)	Wind-cold invasion obstructing the Taiyang channel
	Jiu Wei Qiang Huo Tang* * (Nine Ingredients Qiang Huo Decoction)	Wind-cold-dampness invasion with mild internal heat
	Jia Wei Xiang Su San* * (Augmented Cyperus and Perilla Leaf Powder)	Wind-cold invasion with Qi stagnation

Pungent Warm Exterior Relieving (cont.)	***Xiao Qing Long Tang ***** (Minor Bluegreen Dragon Decoction)	Exterior wind-cold with interior phlegm-fluid retention
	She Gan Ma Huang Tang (Belamcanda and Ephedra Decoction)	Pronounced interior phlegm-fluid with mild exterior condition or without exterior condition
	Jing Fang Bai Du San ** (Schizonepeta and Siler Powder to Overcome Toxicity)	Wind-cold-dampness invasion with strong constitution
Pungent Cool Exterior Relieving 辛凉解表	***Sang Ju Yin ***** (Mulberry Leaf and Chrysanthemum Beverage)	Early stage of wind-heat invasion with mild cough
	Yin Qiao San ** (Lonicera Flower and Forsythia Powder)	Severe wind-heat invasion or early stage of epidemic febrile disease
	Ma Huang Xing Ren Gan Cao Shi Gao Tang ** (Ephedra, Apricot Seed, Licorice, and Gypsum Decoction)	Excessive heat in the lungs from wind-heat invasion or wind-cold turning to heat
	Sheng Ma Ge Gen Tang ** (Cimicifuga and Pueraria Decoction)	Early stage of measles or rashes that do not erupt evenly

Pungent Cool Exterior Relieving (cont.)	***Zhu Ye Liu Bang Tang*** (Bamboo Leaf, Tamarix, and Burdock Seed Decoction)	Early stage of measles with exterior pathogen and interior lung and stomach heat
	Chai Ge Jie Ji Tang ** (Bupleurum and Pueraria Release Muscle Layer Decoction)	Exterior wind-cold or wind-heat with interior heat
	Cong Chi Jie Geng Tang (Scallion, Prepared Soybean, and Platycodon Decoction)	Mild exterior wind-heat and lung heat
	Yue Bi Tang (Maidservant from Yue Decoction)	Initial stage of wind edema with mild heat
Strengthening Body Resistance and Relieving Exterior 扶 正 解 表	***Ren Shen Bai Du San ***** (Ginseng Overcome Toxicity Powder)	Wind-cold-dampness invasion with weakened body resistance(Qi)
	Shen Su Yin (Ginseng and Perilla Leaf Beverage)	Wind-cold invasion with Qi deficiency and phlegm dampness retention
	Zai Zao San ** (Renewal Powder)	Wind-cold invasion with Qi and Yang deficiency

Strengthening Body Resistance and Relieving Exterior (cont.)	*Jia Jian Wei Rui Tang* ** (Modified Polygonatum Decoction)	Wind-heat invasion with Yin deficiency
	Ma Huang Fu Zi Xi Xin Tang (Ephedra, Aconite, and Asarum Decoction)	Invasion of wind-cold with Yang deficiency
Purging Downward with Cold Nature 寒凉泻下	*Da Cheng Qi Tang* ** (Major Decoction for Purging Down Digestive Qi)	Excessive heat accumulating in the Yangming Fu organ
	Xiao Cheng Qi Tang (Minor Decoction for Purging Down Digestive Qi)	Heat accumulating in the Yangming Fu organ
	Tiao Wei Cheng Qi Tang (Regulate Stomach Decoction for Purging Down Digestive Qi)	Mild heat accumulating in the Yangming Fu organ
	Da Xian Xiong Tang (Major Sinking into the Chest Decoction)	Accumulation of heat with phlegm-fluid in the chest and abdomen

Purging Downward with Warm Nature 温热泻下	Da Huang Fu Zi Tang ** (Rhubarb and Prepared Aconite Decoction)	Interior cold accumulation from Yang deficiency
	Wen Pi Tang ** (Warm the Spleen Decoction)	Interior cold accumulation due to deficiency of the spleen Yang
	San Wu Bei Ji Wan (Three Substances for Emergency Pill)	Sudden severe interior excess cold accumulation
Purging Downward with Moist Laxatives 润肠泻下	Ma Zi Ren Wan ** (Hemp Seed Pill)	Pathogenic dry-heat in the Yangming with lack of body fluids
	Run Chang Wan (Moisten the Intestines Pill)	Dryness of the intestines due to Yin or blood deficiency
	Wu Ren Wan (Five Seed Pill)	Lack of body fluid in the intestine or blood deficiency from elderly or postpartum(Mild case)
	Ji Chuan Jian (Benefit the River Decoction)	Constipation in elderly people with kidney Yang, Qi, and essence deficiency

Purging Downward with Harsh Cathartics 峻下逐水	Shi Zao Tang ** Ten Jujube Decoction	Severe interior water retention with strong constitution
	Kong Yan Dan (Control Mucus Elixir)	Phlegm retaining above and below the diaphragm and obstructing Qi
	Zhou Che Wan (Vessel and Vehicle Pill)	Severe interior water and heat accumulation obstructing Qi with strong constitution
	Shu Zuo Yin Zi (Coursing and Piercing Beverage)	Excessive water retention affecting both exterior and interior with strong constitution
Purging Downward with Tonifying Effect 攻补兼施	Xin Jia Huang Long Tang ** (Newly Augmented Yellow Dragon Decoction)	Interior heat accumulation with deficiency of Qi, Yin, and blood
	Zeng Ye Cheng Qi Tang ** (Increase the Fluids and Purge Down Digestive Qi Decoction)	Interior heat accumulation with Yin deficiency

Purging Downward with Tonifying Effect (cont.)	*Huang Long Tang* (Yellow Dragon Decoction)	Interior heat accumulation with Qi and blood deficiency (Stronger purging effect than Xin Jia Huang Long Tang)
Shaoyang Harmonizing 和解少阳	*Xiao Chai Hu Tang* ** (Minor Bupleurum Decoction)	Shaoyang syndrome with pathogen located between exterior and interior
	Hao Qin Qing Dan Tang ** (Sweet Wormwood and Scute Decoction to Clear the Gallbladder)	Damp-heat and turbid-phlegm affecting the gallbladder and Shaoyang channel
	Chai Hu Da Yuan Yin (Bupleurum Beverage to Reach the Primary Membrane)	Epidemic damp-heat complicated with Shaoyang disorder (Malarial disorders)
Regulating the Liver and Spleen (Mediating) 调和肝脾	*Si Ni San* ** (Powder for Treating Cold Limbs)	Internal stagnated Yang Qi which fails to reach the extremities or liver Qi overacting on the stomach
	Chai Hu Shu Gan San ** (Bupleurum Powder to Disperse Liver Qi)	Constraint of the liver Qi with mild blood stagnation

Regulating the Liver and Spleen (Mediating) (cont.)	*Xiao Yao San* ** (Wandering Powder)	Stagnation of the liver Qi with deficiency of the spleen and blood
	Jia Wei Xiao Yao San ** (Augmented Wandering Powder)	Liver Qi stagnation turning to heat with spleen Qi and blood deficiency
	Tong Xie Yao Fang (Important Formula for Painful Diarrhea)	Disharmony between the liver and spleen (Liver Qi overacting on the spleen)
	Shao Yao Gan Cao Tang (Poeny and Licorice Decoction)	Disharmony between the liver and spleen or blood and Yin deficiency with poor circulation
Regulating the Intestines and Stomach (Mediating) 调 和 肠 胃	*Ban Xia Xie Xin Tang* ** (Pinellia Decoction to Purge the Stomach)	Disharmony between the stomach and intestines complicated with cold and heat in the middle burner
	Sheng Jiang Xie Xin Tang (Fresh Ginger Decoction to Purge the Stomach)	Disharmony between the stomach and intestines with water and heat accumulation

Regulating the Intestines and Stomach (Mediating) (cont.)	**Gan Cao Xie Xin Tang** (Licorice Decoction to Purge the Stomach)	Disharmony between the stomach and intestines with stomach Qi deficiency
	Huang Lian Tang (Coptis Decoction)	Upper burner heat and middle burner cold with rebellious stomach Qi
Qi Level Heat Clearing 清气分热	**Bai Hu Tang **** (White Tiger Decoction)	Yangming channel or Qi level excess heat
	Bai Hu Jia Ren Shen Tang (White Tiger Plus Ginseng Decoction)	Yangming channel or Qi level heat with deficiency of Qi and body fluids
	Bai Hu Jia Gui Zhi Tang (White Tiger Plus Cinnamon Decoction)	Heat type of Bi syndrome due to wind-damp-heat invasion
	Zhu Ye Shi Gao Tang ** (Bamboo Leaf and Gypsum Decoction)	Later stage of febrile disease with residual heat in the Qi level and impairment of Qi and body fluids or summer heat damaging the Qi and Yin
Ying and Blood Level Cooling	**Qing Ying Tang **** (Clear the Nutritive Level Decoction)	Heat penetrating into Ying(Nutritive) level

9

清营凉血	**Xi Jiao Di Huang Tang** ** (Rhinoceros Horn and Rehmannia Decoction)	Heat penetrating into blood level
Heat Clearing and Detoxicating 清热解毒	**Huang Lian Jie Du Tang** ** (Coptis Relieve Toxicity Decoction)	Toxic-fire or damp-heat in the three burners
	Xie Xin Tang ** (Drain the Heart Decoction)	Toxic-fire or damp-heat in the upper and middle burners with constipation
	Liang Ge San ** (Cool the Diaphragm Powder)	Excessive fire-heat accumulating in the upper burner and diaphragm
	Pu Ji Xiao Du Yin ** (Universal Benefit Beverage to Relieve Toxicity)	Invasion of seasonal epidemic toxic-heat with wind-heat affecting the head and face
Qi and Blood Level Heat Clearing 气血两清	**Qing Wen Bai Du Yin** ** (Clear Epidemics and Antitoxin Beverage)	Intense epidemic toxic-heat in both Qi and blood levels
Clearing Heat from Zang-fu Organs 清脏腑热	**Dao Chi San** ** (Guide Out the Red Powder)	Heart fire leading to small intestine heat or bladder damp-heat

Clearing Heat from Zang-fu Organs (cont.)	**Qing Xin Lian Zi Yin** (Clear the Heart Beverage with Lotus Seed)	Heart fire and lower burner damp-heat with Qi and Yin deficiency
	Long Dan Xie Gan Tang ** (Gentiana Drain the Liver Decoction)	Liver fire flaring up or liver and gallbladder damp-heat flowing down to lower burner
	Dang Gui Long Hui Wan (Tang-kuei, Gentiana, and Aloe Pill)	Excessive fire in the liver and gallbladder with constipation
	Zuo Jin Wan ** (Left Metal Pill)	Excessive liver fire overacting on the stomach
	Xiang Lian Wan (Aucklandia and Coptis Pill)	Damp-heat in the intestines obstructing Qi (Mild case)
	Xie Bai San ** (Drain the White Powder)	Heat in the lungs
	Ting Li Da Zao Xie Fei Tang (Drain the Lung Decoction with Lepidium and Jujube)	Phlegm-fluid accumulating in the lungs or lung abscess with phlegm
	Qing Wei San ** (Clear the Stomach Powder)	Heat in the stomach

Clearing Heat from Zang-fu Organs (cont.)	**Xie Huang San **** (Drain the Yellow Powder)	Latent fire or damp-heat in the spleen and stomach
	Yu Nu Jian ** (Jade Woman Brew)	Stomach heat with damaged stomach Yin
	Shao Yao Tang ** (Peony Decoction)	Damp-heat in the large intestine with Qi and blood stagnation
	Bai Tou Weng Tang ** (Pulsatilla Decoction)	Large intestine toxic damp-heat penetrating the blood level
	Huang Qin Tang (Scute Decoction)	Heat entering the intestines (Mild case)
Deficient Heat Clearing 清退虚热	**Qing Hao Bie Jia Tang **** (Sweet Wormwood and Turtoise Shell Decoction)	Later stage of febrile disease with latent residual heat and Yin deficiency or chronic disease with damaged Yin
	Qin Jiao Bie Jia San ** (Gentiana Leaf and Tortoise Shell Powder)	Invaded external pathogen turning to heat and hiding in the body with consumption of Yin

Deficient Heat Clearing (cont.)	*Qing Gu San* ** (Clear the Bone-Heat Powder)	Chronic consumptive diseases with severe deficient heat and steaming bone disorder due to Yin deficiency
	Dang Gui Liu Huang Tang (Tang-kuei and Six Yellow Decoction)	Yin deficiency with interior heat causing night sweats
Summer Heat Clearing 祛 署 清 热	*Xin Jia Xiang Ru Yin* ** (Newly Augmented Elsholtzia Beverage)	Early stage of summer heat with externally contracted wind-cold
	Xiang Ru San (Elsholtzia Powder)	Exterior cold with interior dampness in the summer
	Qing Luo Yin (Clear the Collateral Beverage)	Mild summer heat invading the Qi level and lungs
	Liu Yi San ** (Six to One Powder)	Summer heat with dampness
	Qing Shu Yi Qi Tang ** (Clear Summer Heat and Tonify Qi Decoction)	Summer heat with consumption of Qi and Yin

Middle Burner Warming and Cold Dispelling 温中祛寒	Li Zhong Wan ** (Regulate the Middle Burner Pill)	Qi and Yang deficiency of the spleen and stomach with internal cold
	Fu Zi Li Zhong Wan(Tang) {Regulate the Middle Burner Pill(Decoction) with Aconite}	Severe Yang deficiency of the spleen and stomach with internal cold
	Wu Zhu Yu Tang ** (Evodia Decoction)	Deficient cold in the middle burner affecting Jueyin and Shaoyin
	Xiao Jian Zhong Tang ** (Minor Strengthen the Middle Burner Decoction)	Chronic spleen Qi deficiency with spasm in the middle burner due to interior cold (Mild case)
	Huang Qi Jian Zhong Tang (Astragalus Strengthen the Middle Burner Decoction)	Chronic spleen and stomach Qi deficiency with spasm in the middle burner due to interior cold (Severe case)
	Da Jian Zhong Tang ** (Major Strengthen the Middle Burner Decoction)	Spleen Yang deficiency with severe interior cold accumulation

Rescuing Collapsed Yang 回阳救逆	***Si Ni Tang *** (Four Frigid Limbs Decoction)	Severe Yang deficiency of the kidney and spleen with interior cold
	Si Ni Jia Ren Shen Tang (Four Frigid Limbs Decoction with Ginseng)	Yang and Qi collapse with severe blood loss or dehydration
	Tong Mai Si Ni Tang (Unblock the Channel Decoction for Four Frigid Limbs)	Shaoyin syndrome of true cold with false heat
	Shen Fu Tang (Ginseng and Aconite Decoction)	Sudden collapse of Qi and Yang due to loss of blood or severe illness
Channel Warming and Cold Dispelling 温经散寒	***Dang Gui Si Ni Tang *** (Tang-kuei and Four Frigid Limbs Decoction)	Blood deficiency with cold stagnation in the channels
	Huang Qi Gui Zhi Wu Wu Tang (Astragalus and Cinnamon Twig Five Substances Decoction)	Blood stagnation in the channels with Qi deficiency and mild wind invasion
Both Exterior and Interior Relieving	***Da Chai Hu Tang *** (Major Bupleurum Decoction)	Shaoyang disorders with heat accumulating in the Yangming Fu organ

表里双解	**Fang Feng Tong Sheng San **** (Siler Magical Unblocking Powder)	Exterior wind-heat with intense heat in the Qi level and Yangming Fu organ
Both Exterior and Interior Relieving (cont.)	**Ge Gen Huang Qin Huang Lian Tang **** (Pueraria, Scute, and Coptis Decoction)	Exterior wind-heat with large intestine damp-heat
	Chai Hu Gui Zhi Tang (Bupleurum and Cinnamon Twig Decoction)	Shaoyang syndrome with unreleased exterior condition
Qi Tonifying 补气	**Si Jun Zi Tang **** (Four Gentleman Decoction)	Spleen and stomach Qi deficiency
	Liu Jun Zi Tang (Six Gentleman Decoction)	Spleen and stomach Qi deficiency with phlegm-dampness retention
	Xiang Sha Liu Jun Zi Tang (Saussurea, Amomum, and Six Gentleman Decoction)	Spleen and stomach Qi deficiency with dampness obstructing Qi in the middle burner
	Shen Ling Bai Zhu San ** (Ginseng, Hoelen, and White Atractylodes Powder)	Spleen Qi deficiency with severe dampness retention

Qi Tonifying (cont.)	**Bu Zhong Yi Qi Tang** ** (Reinforce the Middle Burner and Tonify Qi Decoction)	Severe deficiency and sinking of spleen and stomach Qi
	Sheng Mai San ** (Activate the Pulse Powder)	Qi and Yin deficiency (Focuses on the heart or lungs)
	Ren Shen Ge Jie San (Ginseng and Gecko Powder)	Lung, spleen, and kidney Qi deficiency with phlegm-dampness and mild heat in the lungs
	Ren Shen Hu Tao Tang (Ginseng and Walnut Decoction)	Lung and kidney Qi deficiency with inability to grasp Qi
	Bu Fei Tang (Tonify the Lungs Decoction)	Lung Qi deficiency with mild lung Yin deficiency
	Sheng Xian Tang (Raise the Sinking Decoction)	Lung and spleen Qi deficiency and sinking
	Ju Yuan Jian (Lift the Source Brew)	Spleen Qi deficiency and sinking
Blood Tonifying	**Si Wu Tang** ** (Four Substances Decoction)	Blood deficiency

补血 **Blood Tonifying (cont.)**	*Tao Hong Si Wu Tang* ** (Four Substances Decoction with Peach Kernel and Safflower)	Blood deficiency with mild blood stagnation
	Bu Gan Tang (Tonify the Liver Decoction)	Liver blood deficiency with mild liver Yin deficiency
Qi and Blood Tonifying 气血双补	*Ba Zhen Tang* ** (Eight Treasure Decoction)	Deficiency of Qi and blood
	Shi Quan Da Bu Tang ** (Great Tonifying Decoction with Ten Ingredients)	Deficiency of Qi and blood with mild deficient cold
	Ren Shen Yang Rong Tang ** (Ginseng Nourish Nutritive Qi Decoction)	Qi, blood, and Yang deficiency with disturbance of spirit
	Tai Shan Pan Shi San (Mount Tai Stabilizing Powder)	Qi and blood deficiency with restless fetus
	Sheng Yu Tang (Sage-like Healing Decoction)	Blood and spleen Qi deficiency with inability to control blood

Qi and Blood Tonifying (cont.)	***Dang Gui Bu Xue Tang*** ** (Tang-kuei Tonify Blood Decoction)	Qi and blood deficiency due to loss of blood with deficient Yang floating to body surface
	Gui Pi Tang ** (Restore the Spleen Decoction)	Heart blood and spleen Qi deficiency or spleen failing to control blood
	Zhi Gan Cao Tang ** (Honey Baked Licorice Decoction)	Blood and Qi deficiency with mild Yin deficiency leading to irregular pulse or consumptive cough (Focus on heart and lungs)
Yin Tonifying 补阴	***Liu Wei Di Huang Wan*** ** (Six Ingredients Pill with Rehmannia)	Yin deficiency of the kidney and liver
	Zhi Bai Di Huang Wan ** (Anemarrhena, Phellodendron, and Rehmannia Pill)	Yin deficiency of the kidney and liver with deficient fire or mild damp-heat in the lower burner.
	Qi Ju Di Huang Wan (Lycium, Chrysanthemum, and Rehmannia Pill)	Yin deficiency of the liver and kidney (Liver deficiency is predominant) with eye disturbance

Yin Tonifying (cont.)	*Du Qi Wan* (Capital Qi Pill)	Yin deficiency of the liver and kidney with mild deficient lung and kidney Qi
	Ba Xian Chang Shou Wan (Eight Immortal Longevity Pill)	Yin deficiency of the lung, liver, and kidney with kidney failing to grasp Qi
	Zuo Gui Wan ** (Left Restoring Pill)	Deficiency of the kidney Yin and essence
	Zuo Gui Yin (Left Restoring Beverage)	Mild deficiency of the kidney and liver Yin
	Da Bu Yin Wan ** (Great Tonify Yin Pill)	Deficiency of the kidney Yin with deficient fire
	Da Bu Yuan Jian (Great Tonify the Primary Brew)	Kidney Yin and Qi deficiency with spleen Qi and blood deficiency
	Jia Jian Fu Mai Tang (Modified Restoring the Pulse Decoction)	Deficiency of Yin and blood with dry heat in the intestines
	Hu Qian Wan ** (The Hidden Tiger Pill)	Yin deficiency of the liver and kidney with deficient fire and weakness of bones and tendons

Yin Tonifying (cont.)	***Er Zhi Wan*** (Two Ultimate Pill)	Mild liver and kidney Yin deficiency with slight deficient heat
	Yi Guan Jian ** (Linking Brew)	Yin deficiency of the liver and kidney with liver Qi stagnation
	Yi Wei Tang (Benefit the Stomach Decoction)	Yin deficiency of the stomach
	Shi Hu Ye Guang Wan (Treat Night Vision Pill with Dendrobium)	Yin deficiency of the liver and kidney with deficient fire and eye disturbance
	Bu Fei E Jiao Tang ** (Tonify the Lungs Decoction with Donkey-hide Gelatin)	Lung Yin deficiency with lung heat
	Yue Hua Wan (Moon Magnificence Pill)	Severe lung and kidney Yin deficiency with dry heat in the lungs
	Gui Lu Er Xian Jiao (Tortoise Plastron and Antler Horn Magic Syrup)	Deficiency of the kidney Yin, Yang, and essence with insufficiency of Qi and blood

Yin Tonifying (cont.)	*Qi Bao Mei Ran Dan* (Seven Treasure Elixir for Beautiful Whiskers)	Yin and essence deficiency of the kidney and deficient liver blood and Yin with early graying hair
	He Che Da Zao Wan (Human Placenta Major Tonifying Pill)	Lung, liver, and kidney Yin deficiency with deficient fire and insufficiency of the kidney essence
	Huang Lian E Jiao Tang (Coptis and Donkey-hide Gelatin Decoction)	Yin deficiency of the heart and kidney with heart fire or later stage of febrile disease affecting the spirit
	Er Dong Tang (Two Winter Decoction)	Diabetes due to Yin and Qi deficiency of the lung and kidney with heat in the upper burner
	Er Long Zuo Ci Wan (Pill for Deafness that is Kind to the Left)	Kidney Yin and essence deficiency with hearing problem
Yang Tonifying 补 阳	*Jin Gui Shen Qi Wan* ** (Tonify Kidney Qi Pill from Golden Cabinet)	Deficiency of the kidney Qi and Yang with decline of Mingmen fire

Yang Tonifying (cont.)	***Ji Sheng Shen Qi Wan*** (Kidney Qi Pill for Aiding the Living)	Deficiency of the kidney Qi and Yang with water retention
	You Gui Wan ** (Right Restoring Pill)	Deficiency of the kidney Yang and essence with decline of Mingmen fire and blood deficiency
	You Gui Yin (Right Restoring Beverage)	Mild deficiency of the kidney Yang and essence
	Wu Bi Shan Yao Wan (Matchless Chinese Wild Yam Pill)	Chronic urinary strengury due to Qi and Yang deficiency of the kidney and spleen
	Nei Bu Wan (Internal Tonification Pill)	Leukorrhea due to kidney Qi and Yang deficiency
Spirit Calming with Heavy Sedative Herbs 重镇安神	***Zhu Sha An Shen Wan ***** (Cinnabar Sedative Pill)	Heart fire flaring up with insufficient heart blood and Yin
	Sheng Tie Luo Yin ** (Iron Filings Beverage)	Manic-depressive disorder due to phlegm-fire disturbing the heart and spirit

Spirit Calming with Heavy Sedative Herbs (cont.)	***Ci Zhu Wan*** (Magnetite and Cinnabar Pill)	Disharmony between kidney water and heart fire with disturbance of spirit
	Zhen Zhu Mu Wan ** (Mother of Pearl Shell Pill)	Yin and blood deficiency of the liver and kidney with raised liver Yang disturbing the spirit
	Chai Hu Jia Long Gu Mu Li Tang (Bupleurum Plus Dragon Bone and Oyster Shell Decoction)	Evil heat invasion from Taiyang into Shaoyang and Yangming with disturbance of spirit and Qi deficiency
Spirit Calming with Nourishing Sedative Herbs 滋养安神	***Suan Zao Ren Tang*** ** (Wild Jujube Seed Decoction)	Deficiency of the liver blood and Yin failing to nourish the heart
	Ding Zhi Wan (Stabilize the Emotions Pill)	Heart Qi deficiency with disturbance of spirit
	Tian Wang Bu Xin Dan ** (Heavenly Emperor Heart Tonifying Elixir)	Deficiency of the heart and kidney Yin and blood with deficient fire flaring up disturbing the spirit

Spirit Calming with Nourishing Sedative Herbs (cont.)	***Bai Zi Yang Xin Wan*** (Biota Seed Nourishing the Heart Pill)	Deficiency of the heart blood and kidney Yin with disturbance of spirit
	Gan Mai Da Zao Tang ** (Licorice, Wheat Chaff, and Jujube Decoction)	Hysteria due to deficiency of the heart and spleen with stagnant liver Qi
	Yang Xin Tang (Nourish the Heart Decoction)	Heart Qi, blood, and Yin deficiency with disturbance of spirit
Aromatically Opening Orifices with Cold Nature 芳香凉开	***An Gong Niu Huang Wan*** ** (Calm the Palace Pill with Ox Gallstone)	Severe epidemic heat penetrating the pericardium or turbid phlegm-heat misting the heart and orifices
	Niu Huang Qing Xin Wan (Clear the Heart Pill with Ox Gallstone)	Heat penetrating the pericardium or phlegm-heat disturbing the spirit
	Zi Xue Dan ** (Purple Snow Elixir)	Epidemic heat penetrating the pericardium with stirring up of the liver wind
	Zhi Bao Dan ** (Greatest Treasure Elixir)	Interior phlegm-heat misting the heart and disturbing the spirit

Aromatically Opening Orifices with Cold Nature (cont.)	***Xiao Er Hui Chun Dan*** (Children Returning Spring Elixir)	Children with excessive phlegm-heat disturbing the spirit and veiling the sensory orifices
Aromatically Opening Orifices with Warm Nature 芳香温开	***Su He Xiang Wan*** ** (Styrax Pill)	Cold phlegm-dampness misting the heart orifices
Consolidating Exterior to Stop Sweating 固表止汗	***Yu Ping Feng San*** ** (Jade Screen Powder)	Deficiency of defensive Qi with spontaneous sweating
	Mu Li San ** (Oyster Shell Powder)	Qi deficiency causing spontaneous and excessive sweating with further injury of heart Yin causing night sweats
Stabilizing the Lungs to Stop Coughing 敛肺止咳	***Jiu Xian San*** (Nine Immortal Powder)	Prolonged cough due to lung Qi and Yin deficiency
Astringing the Intestines to Stop Diarrhea 涩肠止泻	***Zhen Ren Yang Zang Tang*** ** (True Man's Viscera Nourishing Decoction)	Severe Yang deficiency of the spleen and kidney with chronic diarrhea and dysentery

Astringing the Intestines to Stop Diarrhea (cont.)	*Si Shen Wan* ** (Four Miracle Pill)	Deficient cold in the spleen and kidney with dawn diarrhea
	Tao Hua Tang (Peach Blossom Decoction)	Deficient cold in the spleen and stomach with injury to the intestinal collaterals leading to prolonged dysentery
Binding the Essence to Stop Seminal Emission and Enuresis 涩 精 止 遗	*Jin Suo Gu Jing Wan* ** (Golden Lock Essence Stabilizing Pill)	Seminal emission due to deficiency of kidney Yang with inability to consolidate essence
	Shui Lu Er Xian Dan (Water and Land Two Immortals Elixir)	Seminal emission or leukorrhea due to mild insufficiency of the kidney essence and Yang
	Sang Piao Xiao San ** (Praying Mantis Egg-case Powder)	Uncontrolled urine or seminal emission due to Qi and Yin deficiency of the heart and kidney with disharmony and spirit disturbance

Stabilizing the Menses and Stopping Leukorrhea 固 崩 止 带	Gu Jing Wan ** (Stabilize the Menses Pill)	Excessive menses or uterine bleeding due to Yin deficiency with internal heat affecting Chong and Ren channels
	Gu Chong Tang (Stabilize Gushing Decoction)	Spleen Qi deficiency with inability to control blood
	Wan Dai Tang ** (End Discharge Decoction)	Leukorrhea due to spleen Qi deficiency and liver Qi stagnation with dampness retention
	Yi Huang Tang (Change Yellow Decoction)	Leukorrhea due to damp-heat in the lower burner with mild spleen Qi deficiency
Qi Regulating (Moving) 行 气 解 郁	Yue Ju Wan ** (Escape Restraint Pill)	Mild interior stagnancy(blood, phlegm, damp, food, and heat) from restrained liver Qi
	Jin Ling Zi San (Melia Toosandan Powder)	Restrained liver Qi turning to heat with blood stagnation
	Yan Hu Suo San (Corydalis Powder)	Stagnation of blood and Qi due to cold or emotional stress

28

Qi Regulating (Moving) (cont.)	**Ban Xia Hou Pu Tang **** (Pinellia and Magnolia Bark Decoction)	Phlegm and Qi stagnation due to emotional stress with rebellious Qi of the lung and stomach
	Zhi Shi Xie Bai Gui Zhi Tang ** (Immature Bitter Orange, Macrostem Onion, and Cinnamon Twig Decoction)	Phlegm accumulating in the chest with stagnant and rebellious Qi
	Gua Lou Xie Bai Bai Jiu Tang ** (Trichosanthes, Macrostem Onion, and White Wine Decoction)	Phlegm obstructing Yang Qi and blood circulation in the chest
	Gua Lou Xie Bai Ban Xia Tang (Trichosanthes, Macrostem Onion, and Pinellia Decoction)	Severe phlegm accumulation in the chest blocking Qi, blood, and Yang Qi circulation
	Ju He Wan ** (Tangerine Seed Pill)	Stagnation of Qi, blood, and phlegm-damp in the liver channel and lower burner due to damp-cold (Hernia)

Qi Regulating (Moving) (cont.)	*Tian Tai Wu Yao San* ** (Heaven Stage Lindera Powder)	Qi stagnation of the liver channel due to cold invasion (Hernia)
	Nuan Gan Jian ** (Warm the Liver Brew)	Kidney Qi and Yang deficiency with cold stagnation in the liver channel (Hernia)
	Liang Fu Wan (Galanga and Cyperus Pill)	Liver Qi stagnation or cold invasion affecting the stomach
	Hou Po Wen Zhong Tang (Magnolia Bark Decoction to Warm the Middle Burner)	Damp-cold obstructing Qi in the middle burner
	Zheng Qi Tian Xiang San (Qi Correcting Cyperus Powder)	Qi stagnation in the middle burner due to cold
Qi Regulating (Descending) 降气下逆	*Ding Chuan Tang* ** (Arrest Wheezing Decoction)	Phlegm-heat in the lungs or with invasion of wind-cold in the exterior
	Su Zi Jiang Qi Tang ** (Perilla Seed Descending Qi Decoction)	Phlegm-damp in the lungs with Qi and Yang deficiency in the kidney

Qi Regulating (Descending) (cont.)	*Si Mo Tang* ** (Four Milled Herb Decoction)	Emotional upset leading to stagnation of the liver Qi counteracting on the lungs and overacting on the stomach
	Wu Mo Yin Zi (Five Milled Herb Beverage)	Qi stagnation due to severe emotional upset with strong constitution
	Xuan Fu Dai Zhe Tang ** (Elecampane Flower and Hematite Decoction)	Turbid-phlegm accumulation with deficient and rebellious stomach Qi
	Ju Pi Zhu Ru Tang ** (Tangerine Peel and Bamboo Shaving Decoction)	Heat in the stomach with deficient and rebellious stomach Qi
	Ding Xiang Shi Di Tang (Cloves and Kaki Decoction)	Stomach Qi and Yang deficiency with rebellious stomach Qi
Blood Invigorating 活血祛瘀	*Tao He Cheng Qi Tang* ** (Persica Seed Decoction for Purging Down Digestive Qi)	Blood stasis with heat in the lower burner

Blood Invigorating (cont.)	***Xue Fu Zhu Yu Tang** ** (Remove stasis from the Mansion of Blood Decoction)	Blood stasis in the chest with liver Qi stagnation
	Tong Qiao Huo Xue Tang (Unblock the Orifices and Move Blood Decoction)	Blood stasis in the head and face
	***Ge Xia Zhu Yu Tang** ** (Remove Blood Stasis below the Diaphragm Decoction)	Blood stasis below diaphragm with liver Qi stagnation
	***Shao Fu Zhu Yu Tang** ** (Remove Blood Stasis in the Lower Abdomen Decoction)	Blood stasis in the lower burner due to cold
	Shen Tong Zhu Yu Tang (Remove Blood Stasis from Aching Muscle Decoction)	Stagnation of blood and Qi in the channels and collaterals
	***Fu Yuan Huo Xue Tang** ** (Invigorate Blood Decoction for Recovery)	Blood stasis and Qi stagnation in the hypochondrium due to trauma
	Qi Li San (Seven Thousandths of a Tael Powder)	External or internal injury due to trauma with blood stasis and strong constitution

Blood Invigorating (cont.)	***Bu Yang Huan Wu Tang*** ** (Tonify Yang to Restore Five Decoction)	Qi deficiency with blood stasis obstructing the channels
	Shi Xiao San ** (Lose the Smile Powder)	Stagnation of blood in the upper, middle, or lower burner (Mild case)
	Dan Shen Yin ** (Salvia Root Beverage)	Stagnation of blood and Qi in the upper and middle burner (Focus on the heart and stomach)
	Wen Jing Tang ** (Warm the Menses Decoction)	Deficient cold in the Chong and Ren channels with blood stasis and insufficient blood and Yin
	Ai Fu Nuan Gong Wan (Mugwort and Cyperus Pill for Warming the Womb)	Severe deficient cold in the uterus with blood deficiency and mild blood stasis
	Sheng Hua Tang ** (Generating and Transforming Decoction)	Postpartum blood deficiency with blood stagnation due to cold invasion
	Gui Zhi Fu Ling Wan ** (Cinnamon Twig and Hoelen Pill)	Blood stasis and phlegm-dampness accumulating in the uterus

33

Blood Invigorating (cont.)	**Tao Ren Hong Hua Jian** (Peach Kernel and Safflower Brew)	Stagnation of the heart blood with liver Qi stagnation
	Huo Luo Xiao Ling Dan (Effectively Invigorate the Collateral Elixir)	Internal or external blood stasis due to Qi stagnation or trauma
Stopping Bleeding 止 血	**Shi Hui San **** (Ten Charred Ingredients Powder)	Excessive fire-heat in the blood(Focus on liver fire attacking the upper and middle burners)
	Si Sheng Wan (Four Fresh Pill)	Heat in the blood affecting the upper and middle burners (Mild case)
	Ke Xue Fang ** (Coughing of Blood Formula)	Liver fire attacking the lungs with damage of blood vessels
	Huai Hua San ** (Sophora Japonica Flower Powder)	Wind-heat invasion or damp-heat leading to intestinal wind and toxic-heat damaging the blood vessels
	Huai Jiao Wan (Sophora Japonica Fruit Pill)	Wind-heat invasion or toxic damp-heat accumulating in the large intestine causing bleeding hemorrhoids

	Xiao Ji Yin Zi ** (Small Thistle Beverage)	Heat accumulating in the urinary bladder with damaging of blood vessels
Stopping Bleeding (cont.)	Huang Tu Tang ** (Baked Yellow Earth Decoction)	Deficient cold in the middle burner due to spleen Yang and Qi deficiency with inability to control blood
	Jiao Ai Tang ** (Donkey-hide Gelatin and Mugwort Leaf Decoction)	Female bleeding due to imbalance of Chong and Ren channels with Yin and blood deficiency
External Wind Expelling 疏 散 外 风	Da Qin Jiao Tang ** (Large Leaf Gentiana Root Decoction)	External wind-dampness attacking channels and turning to heat with Qi and blood deficiency
	Xiao Feng San ** (Eliminate Wind Powder)	Wind-heat and dampness invasion with pre-existing damp-heat leading to skin disorders
	Chuan Xiong Cha Tiao San ** (Ligusticum Green Tea Mixture)	Headache from externally contracted wind-cold

External Wind Expelling (cont.)	***Cang Er Zi San*** (Xanthium Powder)	Headache and nasal disorders from wind invasion
	Qian Zheng San ** (Pull Straight Powder)	Wind-phlegm attacking the head and facial channels
	Xiao Huo Luo Dan ** (Minor Invigorate the Collateral Elixir)	Wind-cold-dampness or phlegm with blood stasis obstructing the channels and collaterals
	Xiong Zhi Shi Gao Tang (Ligusticum, Angelica Root, and Gypsum Combination)	External wind-heat attacking the collaterals on the head
	Yu Zhen San (Jade Truth Powder)	Tetanus due to wind and toxin invasion through a wound
Internal Wind Extinguish 平熄内风	***Ling Jiao Gou Teng Tang*** ** (Antelope Horn and Uncaria Decoction)	Extreme liver heat stirring up internal wind
	Zhen Gan Xi Feng Tang ** (Sedate the Liver and Extinguish Wind Decoction)	Liver wind stirred up by liver Yang raising due to liver and kidney Yin deficiency

Internal Wind Extinguishing (cont.)	**Tian Ma Gou Teng Yin **** (Gastrodia and Uncaria Beverage)	Liver Yang raising with stirring up liver wind and disturbing the spirit
	E Jiao Ji Zi Huang Tang (Donkey-hide Gelatin and Egg Yolk Decoction)	Endogenous wind due to Yin and blood deficiency with liver Yang raising
	Da Ding Feng Zhu ** (Major Arrest Wind Pearl)	Endogenous wind due to severe Yin and blood deficiency
	Di Huang Yin Zi ** (Rehmannia Beverage)	Kidney Yin and Yang deficiency with phlegm blocking the orifices (Speech disorder)
	San Jia Fu Mai Tang (Three Shells Decoction to Restore the Pulse)	Endogenous wind or liver Yang raising due to Yin and blood deficiency in the later stage of febrile disease or from internal disorders
	Jie Yu Dan (Relieve Slurred Speech Elixir)	Aphasia due to wind-phlegm obstructing the orifices and collaterals

Moistening Dryness 润燥	*Xing Su San* ** (Apricot Seed and Perilla Powder)	External wind-cold and dryness attacking the lungs (Cold dryness)
	Sang Xing Tang ** (Morus and Apricot Seed Decoction)	External wind-heat and dryness attacking the lungs (Warm dryness)
	Qing Zao Jiu Fei Tang ** (Clear Dryness and Rescue the Lung Decoction)	Dry heat attacking the lungs with damage of lung Yin and mild injury of lung Qi
	Sha Shen Mai Men Dong Tang (Glehnia and Ophiopogon Decoction)	Lung and stomach Yin deficiency due to dry heat
	Yang Yin Qing Fei Tang ** (Nourish Yin and Clear the Lung Decoction)	Diphtheria with lung Yin deficiency
	Bai He Gu Jin Tang ** (Lily Bulb Decoction to Consolidate the Metal)	Lung and kidney Yin deficiency with deficient heat
	Mai Men Dong Tang ** (Ophiopogon Decoction)	Insufficiency of the lung and stomach Yin with rebellious and deficient Qi

Moistening Dryness (cont.)	**Zeng Ye Tang** (Increase the Fluids Decoction)	Yin deficiency with dry heat in the Yangming system
Dampness Drying and Stomach Harmonizing 燥湿和胃	**Ping Wei San **** (Calm the Stomach Powder)	Dampness obstructing Qi in the spleen and stomach
	Huo Xiang Zheng Qi San ** (Agastache Qi Rectifying Powder)	External wind-cold with internal dampness obstructing Qi in the middle burner
	Bu Huan Jin Zheng Qi San (Qi Rectifying Powder Worth More Than Gold)	External wind-cold with turbid dampness attacking the stomach and intestines
Damp-heat Clearing 清热祛湿	**Yin Chen Hao Tang **** (Capillaris Decoction)	Yang Jaundice due to damp-heat
	San Ren Tang ** (Three Seeds Decoction)	External or internal damp-heat (Dampness is predominant) obstructing in the Qi level
	Huo Pu Xia Ling Tang (Agastache, Magnolia, Pinellia, and Poria Decoction)	Wind-damp-heat invasion with internal dampness retention

Damp-heat Clearing (cont.)	**Gan Lu Xiao Du Dan **** (Sweet Dew Toxin Eliminating Elixir)	Toxic damp-heat or seasonal epidemic damp-heat retaining in the Qi level
	Ba Zheng San ** (Eight Straight Powder)	Damp-heat in the urinary bladder
	Er Miao San ** (Two Mysterious Powder)	Damp-heat in the lower burner
	San Miao Wan (Three Mysterious Pill)	Damp-heat in the lower burner with weakness of bone and tendon
	Si Miao Wan (Four Mysterious Pill)	Damp-heat in the lower burner with predominant dampness and weakness of bone and tendon
	Bei Xie Fen Qing Yin II** (Hypoglauca Yam Beverage to Separate Clear from Turbid)	Turbid damp-heat in the lower burner with cloudy urine
	Fu Ling Pi Tang (Hoelen Peel Decoction)	Damp-heat in the middle and lower burner
	Shi Wei San (Pyrrosia Leaf Powder)	Damp-heat in the urinary bladder with stones

Downward Dampness Draining 利水渗湿	***Wu Ling San*** ****** (Five Ingredients Powder with Poria)	Water retention with spleen Qi deficiency or mild wind-cold in the exterior
	Yin Chen Wu Ling San ****** (Five Ingredients Powder with Poria plus Capillaris)	Yang jaundice due to damp-heat with pronounced dampness
	Wei Ling Tang ****** (Stomach Calming and Hoelen Five Decoction)	Pronounced dampness accumulating in the middle burner with Qi stagnation
	Zhu Ling Tang ****** (Polyporus Decoction)	Water accumulating in the lower burner with heat and injured Yin
	Fang Ji Huang Qi Tang (Stephania and Astragalus Decoction)	Wind-damp edema with spleen and defensive Qi deficiency
	Wu Pi San(Yin) (Five Peel Powder)	Dampness retention with stagnant Qi and mild spleen Qi deficiency
Yang Warming and Dampness Transforming	***Ling Gui Zhu Gan Tang*** ****** (Poria, Cinnamon, Atracthlodes, and Licorice Decoction)	Phlegm-fluid retention affecting the upper or middle burner with spleen Yang deficiency

温化水湿	*Zhen Wu Tang* ** (True Warrior Decoction)	Water retention with Yang deficiency of the heart, spleen, and kidney
Yang Warming and Dampness Transforming (cont.)	*Shi Pi San(Yin)* ** (Bolster the Spleen Powder)	Spleen and kidney Yang deficiency with water retention and stagnant Qi (Yin edema)
	Bei Xie Fen Qing Yin I (Hypoglauca Yam Beverage to Separate the Clear from Turbid)	Damp-cold in the lower burner with kidney Qi and Yang deficiency causing cloudy urine
Wind-dampness Expelling 祛风胜湿	*Qiang Huo Sheng Shi Tang* ** (Notopterygium Decoction to Overcome Dampness)	Wind-dampness invading the superficial channels
	Juan Bi Tang ** (Alleviating Painful Obstruction Decoction)	Painful Bi syndrome due to wind-dampness invasion with Qi deficiency
	Du Huo Ji Sheng Tang ** (Pubescent Angelica and Loranthus Decoction)	Chronic Bi syndrome due to wind-cold-dampness invasion with deficiency of the liver, kidney, Qi and blood

Wind-dampness Expelling (cont.)	***San Bi Tang*** (Three Painful Obstruction Decoction)	Chronic Bi syndrome due to wind-dampness invasion with Qi and blood deficiency and weakness of the liver and kidney
	Ji Ming San (Powder to Take at Cock's Crow)	Damp-cold obstructing in the channels of lower limbs causing beriberi
	Fang Feng Tang (Ledebouriella Decoction)	Wind-cold-damp Bi syndrome with predominant wind
	Wu Tou Tang (Aconite Decoction)	Wind-cold-damp Bi syndrome with predominant cold and weakness of Qi
Dampness Drying and Phlegm Resolving 燥湿化痰	***Er Chen Tang ***** (Two Matured Ingredients Decoction)	Phlegm-dampness obstructing the Qi in the upper and middle burners
	Dao Tan Tang (Guide Out Phlegm Decoction)	Excessive phlegm-dampness obstructing Qi, affecting the lungs, or misting the orifices

Dampness Drying and Phlegm Resolving (cont.)	*Di Tan Tang* (Phlegm Flushing Decoction)	Phlegm misting the heart and orifices or with internal liver wind
	Wen Dan Tang ** (Warm the Gallbladder Decoction)	Disharmony between the gallbladder and stomach with phlegm-heat
Heat Clearing and Phlegm Resolving 清热化痰	*Qing Qi Hua Tan Wan* ** (Clear Qi and Resolve Phlegm Pill)	Mild phlegm-heat in the lungs
	Xiao Xian Xiong Tang ** (Minor Sinking into Chest Decoction)	Phlegm-heat accumulating in the chest and epigastrium
	Gun Tan Wan (Rolling Out Phlegm Pill)	Phlegm-fire disturbing the heart and orifices
	Sang Bai Pi Tang (Mulberry Rootbark Decoction)	Phlegm-heat in the lungs
	Qing Jin Hua Tan Tang (Clear Metal and Resolve Phlegm Decoction)	Phlegm-heat in the lungs with mild damage of lung Yin
Dryness Moistening and Phlegm Resolving 润燥化痰	*Bei Mu Gua Lou San* ** (Fritillary and Trichosanthes Fruit Powder)	Dry-phlegm in the lungs with mild injury to Yin

Cold-Phlegm Transforming 温化寒痰	*Ling Gan Wu Wei Jiang Xin Tang* (Poria, Licorice, Schisandra, Ginger, and Asarum Decoction)	Cold phlegm-fluid retaining in the lungs with spleen Yang deficiency
	San Zi Yang Qin Tang ** (Three Seeds Nourishing the Parents Decoction)	Cold-phlegm in the lungs with Qi and food stagnation
Treating Wind-phlegm 治风化痰	*Ban Xia Bai Zhu Tian Ma Tang* ** (Pinellia, White Atractylodes, and Gastrodia Decoction)	Up-stirring of the liver wind with phlegm
	Ding Xian Wan ** (Stabilizing Epilepsy Pill)	Liver wind with phlegm-heat leading to recurrent seizures
	Zhi Sou San ** (Relieving Cough Powder)	External wind invading the lungs with internal phlegm
Food Stagnation Relieving 消导化积	*Bao He Wan* ** (Preserving Harmony Pill)	Mild food stagnation
	Zhi Shi Dao Zhi Wan ** (Guide Out Stagnation with Immature Bitter Orange Pill)	Food stagnation with damp-heat retention

Food Stagnation Relieving (cont.)	***Mu Xiang Bing Lang Wan*** ** (Aucklandia and Betel Nut Pill)	Severe food and Qi stagnation with damp-heat retention
	Zhi Zhu Wan ** (Immature Bitter Orange and Atractylodes Pill)	Mild spleen Qi deficiency with Qi and food stagnation
	Jian Pi Wan ** (Strengthen the Spleen Pill)	Severe spleen and stomach Qi deficiency with food stagnation
	Zhi Shi Xiao Pi Wan (Immature Bitter Orange Pill to Relieve Focal Distention)	Spleen Qi deficiency with Qi/food stagnation and complicated cold/heat signs
Parasites Expelling 驱虫	***Wu Mei Wan*** ** (Mume Pill)	Roundworm disturbance due to upper(Stomach) heat and lower(Intestines) cold with deficiency of Qi and blood
	Li Zhong An Hui Tang (Regulate the Middle and Calm Roundworms Decoction)	Deficient cold in the spleen and stomach with roundworm disturbance

Parasites Expelling (cont.)	*Fei Er Wan* ** (Fat Baby Pill)	Malnutrition due to parasites accumulation with spleen deficiency and stomach heat
Inducing Vomiting 涌吐	*Gua Di San* ** (Melon Pedicle Powder)	Phlegm and food retention obstructing in the chest and epigastrium
Treating External Carbuncles 治外疡	*Xian Fang Huo Ming Yin* ** (Celestial Formula for Sustaining Life Beverage)	Early stage of carbuncles and boils with toxic phlegm-fire and stagnation of Qi and blood
	Wu Wei Xiao Du Yin ** (Five Ingredients Beverage to Relieve Toxin)	Carbuncles, boils, and sores due to toxic-fire contracted externally or produced by dysfunction of Zang-fu organs
	Si Miao Yong An Tang ** (Four Mysterious Ingredients Decoction for Calming Hero)	Gangrene due to toxic heat and blood stagnation
	Niu Bang Jie Ji Tang (Burdock Seed Release Muscle Decoction)	Localized carbuncles and boils due to toxic phlegm-heat accompanied with exterior wind-heat

Treating External Carbuncles (cont.)	*Hai Zao Yu Hu Tang* ** (Sargassum Jade Flask Decoction)	Qi Goiter due to disharmony between the liver and spleen with stagnation of phlegm, dampness, Qi, and blood
	Tou Nong San ** (Discharge Pus Powder)	Chronic carbuncles and boils with deficiency of Qi and blood
	Yang He Tang ** (Yang Harmony Decoction)	Carbuncles due to cold-phlegm obstruction with Yang and blood deficiency
Treating Internal Abscesses 治内痈	*Wei Jing Tang* ** (Reed Decoction)	Toxic phlegm-heat and stagnant blood in the lungs
	Da Huang Mu Dan Tang ** (Rhubarb and Moutan Decoction)	Intestinal abscess due to toxic damp-heat and stagnant blood in the intestines
	Yi Yi Fu Zi Bai Jiang San (Coix, Aconite, and Baijiang Powder)	Intestinal abscess with formation of pus due to damp-cold and stagnant blood
	Yi Yi Ren Tang (Coix Seed Decoction)	Early stage of intestinal abscess with dampness retention and stagnant blood

Additional Formulas for Internal Medicine 内 科 附 方	**_Ji Jiao Li Huang Wan_** (Stephania, Zanthoxylum, Lepidium, and Rhubarb Pill)	Edema with constipation due to accumulated heat and water obstructing Qi in the stomach and large intestine
	Zhong Man Fen Xiao Wan (Middle Burner Fullness Separating and Reducing Pill)	Drum distention(Gu Zhang) due to damp-heat obstructing in the middle burner with underlying spleen Qi deficiency
	Wu Zi Yan Zong Wan ** (Five Seed Progeny Pill)	Reproductive disorders due to kidney Qi, Yang, and essence deficiency
	Jiao Tai Wan (Grand Communication Pill)	Disharmony between the heart and kidney
	He Ren Yin (Fleece Flower and Ginseng Pill)	Chronic malaria with liver blood and spleen Qi deficiency
	Gui Zhi Gan Cao Long Gu Mu Li Tang (Cinnamon, Licorice, Dragon Bone, and Oyster Shell Decoction)	Palpitation and disturbed spirit due to heart Yang and Yin deficiency caused by Taiyang disease, excessive sweating, or inappropriate using of warming herbs

Additional Formulas for Internal Medicine (cont.)	*Xiao Ke Fang* ****** (Wasting Thirst Formula)	Upper burner pattern of diabetes with lung heat and damage of Yin fluids
	Liu Mo Tang (Six Milled Herbs Decoction)	Constipation due to Qi stagnation
	Huang Qi Tang (Astragalus Decoction)	Constipation due to Qi deficiency
	Yin Chen Zhu Fu Tang (Oriental Wormwood, Atractylodes, and Aconite Decoction)	Yin jaundice due to damp-cold and spleen Yang deficiency
	Gan Jiang Ling Zhu Tang (Licorice, Dried Ginger, Hoelen, and Atractylodes Decoction)	Lower back pain due to invaded damp-cold obstructing in the channels and collaterals
	San Cai Feng Sui Dan (Three-talent Retaining Marrow Elixir)	Seminal emission due to kidney Yin deficiency with exuberant deficient fire
Additional Formulas for Ob-Gyn Disorders 妇产科附方	*Xia Ru Yong Quan San* ****** (Promoting Lactation and Gushing Spring Powder)	Insufficient lactation due to liver Qi stagnation

妇产科附方	**Tong Ru Dan** ** (Promote Lactation Elixir)	Insufficient lactation due to deficiency of Qi and blood
Additional Formulas for Ob-Gyn Disorders (cont.)	**Su Ye Huang Lian Tang** (Perilla Leaf and Coptis Decoction)	Morning sickness due to disharmony between the liver and stomach
	Shou Tai Wan ** (Fetus Longevity Pill)	Threatened miscarriage due to kidney Qi deficiency
	Tai Yuan Yin (Fetal Origin Beverage)	Threatened miscarriage due to deficiency of Qi and blood
	Qing Jing San (Channel Clearing Powder)	Antedated menstruation due to excess heat in the blood
	Zhi Dai Fang (Stopping Discharge Formula)	Leukorrhea due to downward flowing of damp-heat
	Gu Ben Zhi Beng Tang ** (Secure Root and Stop Uterine Bleeding Decoction)	Uncontrolled uterine bleeding due to spleen Qi deficiency
	Qing Re Gu Jing Tang ** (Clear Heat and Secure Menses Decoction)	Severe uterine bleeding due to excess heat in the blood

Additional Formulas for Ob-Gyn Disorders (cont.)	***Bei Xie Shen Shi Tang*** (Hypoglauca Yam Dampness Draining Decoction)	Vaginal itching due to downward flowing of damp-heat in the liver channel
	She Chuang Zi San (Cnidium Seed Powder)	Externally used formula for vaginal itching due to toxic damp-heat
	Yang Jing Zhong Yu Tang ** (Nourish Essence and Plant Jade Decoction)	Infertility due to kidney Yin and essence deficiency
	Kai Yu Zhong Yu Tang (Open Depression and Plant Jade Decoction)	Infertility due to liver Qi stagnation
	Er Xian Tang ** (Two Immortals Decoction)	Pre and post menopausal syndrome or chronic diseases with kidney Yin, Yang, and essence deficiency

Ai Fu Nuan Gong Wan-Mugwort and Cyperu Pill for Warming the Womb

艾附暖宮丸

■ **Ingredients**

Ai Ye	Mugwort Leaf	90g
Xiang Fu	Cyperus Tuber	180g
Wu Zhu Yu	Evodia	90g
Chuan Xiong	Ligusticum	60g
Bai Shao Yao	White Peony	90g
Huang Qi	Astragalus	90g
Xu Duan	Teasel Root	45g
Sheng Di Huang	Dried Rehmannia	30g
Rou Gui	Cinnamon Bark	15g
Dang Gui	Chinese Angelica	90g

■ **Preparation**

Use as prepared form or decoction with properly reduced dosage.

■ **Pertaining Category**

Blood Invigorating

■ **Functions**

Warms the uterus and channels, nourishes blood, regulates menses, calms the fetus.

■ **Indications**

Severe deficient cold in the uterus with blood deficiency and slight blood stasis manifested as prolonged menstrual duration, or intermittent lower abdominal cold pain and distention during pregnancy, or failure to conceive for long time, watery clear vaginal discharge, pale or sallow complexion, cold and painful limbs, lassitude, poor appetite, irregular menstruation, pale tongue with white coat, a frail pulse

■   **Cautions and Contraindications**
None noted.

■   **Modern Applications**
Irregular menstruation, dysmenorrhea, infertility, leukorrhea,
threatened abortion, etc.
*Shu Di Huang(Cooked Rehmannia) can be used instead of Sheng
Di Huang according to the condition of the patient.*

An Gong Niu Huang Wan-Calm the Palace
Pill with Ox Gallstone
Ox Gallstone and Curcuma Formula
安 宫 牛 黄 丸

■   **Ingredients**

Niu Huang	*Ox Gallstone*	30g
Yu Jin	*Curcuma Root*	30g
Xi Jiao	*Rhinoceros Horn*	30g
Huang Lian	*Coptis*	30g
Huang Qin	*Scute*	30g
Zhi Zi	*Gardenia*	30g
Zhu Sha	*Cinnabar*	30g
Xiong Huang	*Realgar*	30g
Bing Pian	*Borneol*	7.5g
She Xiang	*Musk*	7.5g
Zhen Zhu	*Pearl*	15g

■   **Preparation**
Use as prepared form only.

■   **Pertaining Category**
Opening Orifices with Cold Nature

■ Functions

Clears heat, relieves toxicity. Eliminates phlegm, opens orifices, induces resuscitation.

■ Indications

Epidemic febrile diseases with heat penetrating the pericardium or phlegm heat disturbing the heart manifested as high fever, restlessness, delirium, impaired spirit, loss of consciousness or coma due to stroke, or infantile convulsion, dark red tongue with yellow greasy coat, a wiry, and forceful pulse.

■ Cautions and Contraindications

It is contraindicated in cases of coma due to cold phlegm and during pregnancy. Do not use for long term.

■ Modern Applications

Encephalitis B, epidemic cerebral-spinal meningitis, cerebral vascular accident, urimia, toxic pneumonia, toxic dysentery, hepatic coma, infantile convulsions, etc.

Ba Xian Chang Shou Wan-Eight Immortal Longevity Pill
Ophiopogon, Schizandra, and Rehmannia Pill
八仙长寿丸 (麦味地黄丸)

■ Ingredients

Shu Di Huang	Cooked Rehmanni	24g
Shan Zhu Yu	Dogwood Fruit	12g
Shan Yao	Dioscorea	12g
Fu Ling	Hoelen/Poria	9g
Ze Xie	Alisma	9g
Mu Dan Pi	Moutan Bark	9g
Mai Men Dong	Ophiopogon	9g
Wu Wei Zi	Schizandra	6g

■ **Preparation**
Use as decoction or prepared form.

■ **Pertaining Category**
Yin Tonifying

■ **Functions**
Nourishes the kidney, liver, and lung Yin, astrigents the Qi, stops coughing and wheezing.

■ **Indications**
Yin deficiency of the lungs and kidneys manifested as cough, wheezing, difficulty in breathing, worse in the afternoon, weak voice, shortness of breath, soreness and weakness of lower back, tidal fever, night sweats, or nocturnal emission, red tongue with scanty coat, a thin, rapid pulse.

■ **Cautions and Contraindications**
Use with extreme caution for patients with indigestion, diarrhea due to deficiency of the spleen and stomach.

■ **Modern Applications**
Chronic cough, asthma, hemoptysis, pulmonary emphysema, pulmonary tuberculosis, diabetes, etc.

Ba Zhen Tang-Eight Treasure Decoction
Tang-kuei and Ginseng Eight Combination
八珍汤

■   **Ingredients**

Dang Gui	Chinese Angelica	10g
Chuan Xiong	Ligusticum	5g
Bai Shao Yao	White Peony	8g
Shu Di Huang	Cooked Rehmannia	15g
Ren Shen	Ginseng	3-6g
Bai Zhu	White Atractylodes	10g
Fu Ling	Hoelen/Poria	8g
Zhi Gan Cao	Baked Licorice	5g
Sheng Jiang	Fresh Ginger	3slices
Da Zao	Jujube	2pcs

■   **Preparation**
Use as decoction or prepared form.

■   **Pertaining Category**
Qi and Blood Tonifying

■   **Functions**
Tonifies Qi, nourishes blood, strengthens the spleen.

■   **Indications**
Deficiency of Qi and blood manifested as pale or sallow complexion
dizziness, blurred vision, lassitude, shortness of breath, weak voice,
dislike to speak, palpitation, poor appetite, pale tongue with thin
white coat, a thin, weak pulse.

■   **Cautions and Contraindications**
None noted.

■   **Modern Applications**
Anemia, irregular menstruation, chronic diseases, post-surgical
recovery, neurasthenia, etc.

Ba Zheng San-Eight Straight Powder
Dianthus Formula
八 正 散

■   **Ingredients**

Qu Mai	Dianthus	6-12g
Che Qian Zi	Plantago Seed	6-9g
Bian Xu	Polygonum	6-9g
Hua Shi	Talcum	12-18g
Zhi Zi	Gardenia Fruit	6-9g
Mu Tong	Akebia Stem	6-9g
Da Huang	Rhubarb	6-9g
Deng Xin Cao	Rush Pith	3-6g
Zhi Gan Cao	Baked Licorice	3-6g

■   **Preparation**

Use as decoction or prepared form. Che Qian Zi should be wrapped in gauze when making decoction.

■   **Pertaining Category**

Damp-heat Clearing

■   **Functions**

Clears heat, purges fire. Promotes urination, unblocks urinary strangury.

■   **Indications**

Damp-heat in the urinary bladder manifested as spasmodic, distending pain in the lower abdomen and lower back, frequent dark, scanty, painful, difficult or cloudy urination with ergency, or retention of urine, dry mouth and throat, red tongue with yellow coat, a slippery, rapid, and forceful pulse.

■ **Cautions and Contraindications**

It is contraindicated for pregnant women and patients with weak constitution. Do not use overdose and for long term.

■ **Modern Applications**

Acute UTI, cystitis, pyelitis, pyelonephritis, urinary tract calculi, prostatitis,etc.

Bai He Gu Jin Tang-Lily Bulb Decoction to Consolidate the Metal
Lily Combination
百 合 固 金 汤

■ **Ingredients**

Sheng Di Huang	*Dried Rehmannia*	6g
Shu Di Huang	*Cooked Rehmannia*	9g
Mai Men Dong	*Ophiopogon*	5g
Bai He	*Lily Bulb*	3g
Bai Shao Yao	*White Peony*	3g
Chuan Bei Mu	*Tendrilled Fritillary*	3g
Dang Gui	*Chinese Angelica*	3g
Xuan Shen	*Scrophularia Root*	3g
Jie Geng	*Platycodon*	3g
Gan Cao	*Licorice*	3g

■ **Preparation**

Use as decoction or prepared form.

■ **Pertaining Category**

Moistening Dryness

■ **Functions**

Nourishes Yin, moistens the lungs. Clears heat, cools blood. Resolves phlegm, stops coughing.

■ Indications

Lung and kidney Yin deficiency with deficient heat manifested as dry and sore throat, cough with blood-tinged sputum, difficult breathing, a feverish sensation in the palms and soles, or night sweats, red tongue with scanty coat, a thin, rapid pulse.

■ Cautions and Contraindications

It is contraindicated in cases of diarrhea, abdominal distention and pain, poor appetite due to spleen deficiency.

■ Modern Applications

Pulmonary tuberculosis, bronchietasis, chronic laryngopharyngitis, chronic bronchitis, etc.

Bai Hu Jia Gui Zhi Tang-White Tiger Plus Cinnamon Decoction
Cinnamon and Gypsum Combination
白 虎 加 桂 枝 汤

■ Ingredients

Shi Gao	Gypsum	30g
Zhi Mu	Anemarrhena	9g
Zhi Gan Cao	Baked Licorice	3g
Geng Mi	Oryza	6g
Gui Zhi	Cinnamon Twig	9g

■ Preparation

Use as decoction or prepared form.

■ Pertaining Category

Qi Level Heat Clearing

■ Functions

Clears heat, promotes generation of body fluids. Harmonizes nutritive and defensive Qi. Removes obstruction of channels and collaterals.

■ Indications

Heat bi syndrome due to wind-damp-heat invasion or wind-damp turning to heat manifested as high fever, coarse breathing, irritability, thirst, swelling and painful joints with heat sensation. Also used for warm malarial disorder with intense fever and mild chills, or no chills, aching joints, occasional vomiting, white or yellow tongue coat, a wiry, rapid pulse.

■ Cautions and Contraindications

It is contraindicated in cases of fever due to Yin and blood deficiency, or pattern of true cold with false heat.

■ Modern Applications

Rheumatic arthritis, rheumatism, malaria, etc.
This formula is modified from Bai Hu Tang (White Tiger Decoction).

Bai Hu Jia Ren Shen Tang-White Tiger Plus Ginseng Decoction
Ginseng and Gypsum Combination
白 虎 加 人 参 汤

■ Ingredients

Shi Gao	Gypsum	30g
Zhi Mu	Anemarrhena	9g
Zhi Gan Cao	Baked Licorice	3g
Geng Mi	Cryza	9g
Ren Shen	Ginseng	9g

- **Preparation**

Use as decoction or prepared form.

- **Pertaining Category**

Qi Level Heat Clearing

- **Functions**

Clears heat in the Qi level, promotes the generation of body fluid. Tonifies Qi.

- **Indications**

Yangming channel or Qi level heat with deficiency of Qi and body fluids or summer heat with consumption of Qi and Yin manifested as fever, thirst, severe sweating, slight aversion to cold in the back, red tongue with yellow dry coat, a flooding, rapid, and forceless pulse.

- **Cautions and Contraindications**

It is contraindicated in cases of unrelieved exterior syndrome, fever due to blood and yin deficiency, and pattern of true cold with false heat.

- **Modern Applications**

Influenza, epidemic encephalitis, epidemic meningitis, pneumonia, septicemia, gingivitis, etc.

Bai Hu Tang-White Tiger Decoction
Gypsum Combination
白 虎 汤

- **Ingredients**

Shi Gao	*Gypsum*	30g
Zhi Mu	*Anemarrhena*	9g
Zhi Gan Cao	*Baked Licorice*	3g
Geng Mi	*Oryza*	9g

■ Preparation
Use as decoction or prepared form.

■ Pertaining Category
Qi Level Heat Clearing

■ Functions
Clears heat in the Qi level, drains stomach fire. Promotes the generation of body fluids.

■ Indications
Yangming channel or Qi level excess heat manifested as high fever red flushed complexion, excessive sweating, aversion to heat, irritability, thirst with a strong desire to drink, red tongue with yellow dry coat, a flooding, rapid, forceful, or slippery, rapid pulse.

■ Cautions and Contraindications
It is contraindicated in cases of unrelieved exterior syndrome, fever due to blood and Yin deficiency, and pattern of true cold with false heat.

■ Modern Applications
Influenza, epidemic encephalitis, epidemic meningitis, pneumonia, septicemia, gingivitis, etc.

Bai Tou Weng Tang-Pulsatilla Decoction
Pulsatilla Combination
白头翁汤

■ Ingredients

Bai Tou Weng	*Pulsatilla*	15g
Huang Bai	*Phellodendron*	12g
Huang Lian	*Coptis*	6g
Qin Pi	*Fraxinus*	12g

■ Preparation
Use as decoction or prepared form.

■ **Pertaining Category**
Clearing Heat from Zang-fu Organs

■ **Functions**
Clears damp-heat, relieves toxicity. Cools blood, stops dysentery.

■ **Indications**
Large intestine toxic damp-heat penetrating the blood level marked by more blood and less mucus in the stools, abdominal pain with tenesmus, a burning sensation in the anus, feverish body, irritability thirst with desire to drink, red tongue with yellow coat, a rapid pulse.

■ **Cautions and Contraindications**
It is contraindicated in cases of dysentery of chronic and deficient types.

■ **Modern Applications**
Acute dysentery, acute enteritis, amebic dysentery, ulcerative colitis, etc.

Bai Zi Yang Xin Wan-Biota Seed Nourishing the Heart Pill
柏子养心丸

■ **Ingredients**

Bai Zi Ren	Biota Seed	120g
Gou Qi Zi	Lycium Fruit	90g
Mai Men Dong	Ophiopogon	30g
Dang Gui	Chinese Angelica	30g
Xuan Shen	Scrophularia	60g
Shu Di Huang	Cooked Rehmanni	60g
Shi Chang Pu	Sweetflag Rhizome	30g
Fu Shen	Hoelen/Poria	30g
Gan Cao	Licorice	15g

- **Preparation**

Use as prepared form or decoction with properly reduced dosage.

- **Pertaining Category**

Spirit Calming with Nourishing Sedative Herbs

- **Functions**

Nourishes the heart blood and kidney Yin, calms spirit.

- **Indications**

Deficiency of the heart blood and kidney Yin manifested as disorientation, palpitation, insomnia, dream disturbed sleep, dizziness, poor memory, night sweats, slight red or pale tongue with scanty coat, a thin, or thin, rapid pulse.

- **Cautions and Contraindications**

None noted.

- **Modern Applications**

Cardiac neurosis, paroxysmal tachycardia, neurasthenia, insomnia, etc.

Ban Xia Bai Zhu Tian Ma Tang-Pinellia, White Atractylodes, and Gastrodia Decoction
Pinellia and Gastrodia Combination
半夏白术天麻汤

- **Ingredients**

Ban Xia	*Pinellia Tuber*	9g
Bai Zhu	*White Atractylodes*	15g
Tian Ma	*Gastrodia*	6g
Fu Ling	*Hoelen/Poria*	6g
Chen Pi	*Tangerine Peel*	6g
Sheng Jiang	*Fresh Ginger*	1 slice
Da Zao	*Jujube*	2 pcs
Gan Cao	*Licorice*	4g

- **Preparation**

Use as decoction or prepared form.

- **Pertaining Category**

Treating Wind-phlegm

- **Functions**

Dries dampness, resolves phlegm, strengthens the spleen. Calms the liver, extinguishes the endogenous wind.

- **Indications**

Up-stirring of liver wind with phlegm manifested as dizziness, vertigo, headache, fullness sensation in the chest, copious sputum, nausea, vomiting, poor appetite, or lethargy, deviation of the eyes and mouth, white greasy tongue coat, a wiry, slippery pulse.

- **Cautions and Contraindications**

It is contraindicated in cases of dizziness and headache due to liver Yang raising caused by liver and kidney Yin deficiency or blood deficiency.

- **Modern Applications**

Pulmonary emphysema, Meniere's syndrome, dysfunction of vegetative (autonomic) nerve, cerebral arteriosclerosis, hypertension, benign positional vertigo, etc.

Ban Xia Hou Po Tang-Pinellia and Magnolia Bark Decoction
半夏厚朴汤

- **Ingredients**

Ban Xia	Pinellia Tuber	12g
Hou Po	Magnolia Bark	9g
Fu Ling	Hoelen/Poria	12g
Zi Su Ye	Perilla Leaf	6g
Sheng Jiang	Fresh Ginger	9-15g

■ Preparation
Use as decoction or prepared form.

■ Pertaining Category
Qi Regulating (Moving)

■ Functions
Moves Qi, resolves phlegm, and disperses lumps. Descends the adverse flow of Qi.

■ Indications
Phlegm and Qi stagnation manifested as a blocking sensation in the throat as if a plum pit is stuck in the throat which is difficulty in swallowing down or vomiting out, a fullness sensation in the chest or hypochondrium, cough with white sputum, or nausea, white greasy moist tongue coat, a wiry, slippery pulse.

■ Cautions and Contraindications
It is contraindicated in cases of lack of body fluid or Yin deficiency with deficient fire.

■ Modern Applications
Hysteria, pharyngoneurosis, chronic pharyngitis or laryngitis, asthma, neurogenic vomiting, gastric neurosis, morning sickness, etc.

Ban Xia Xie Xin Tang-Pinellia Decoction to Purge the Stomach
Pinellia Combination
半夏泻心汤

■ Ingredients

Ban Xia	Pinellia Tuber	9g
Huang Qin	Scute	6g
Gan Jiang	Dried Ginger	6g
Ren Shen	Ginseng	6g
Huang Lian	Coptis	3g
Zhi Gan Cao	Baked Licorice	6g
Da Zao	Jujube	4pcs

■ Preparation
Use as decoction or prepared form.

■ Pertaining Category
Regulating the Intestine and Stomach (Mediating).

■ Functions
Harmonizes the stomach, descends the rebellious stomach Qi.
Regulates the stomach and intestines, relieves focal distention.

■ Indications
Disharmony between the stomach and intestines complicated with cold and heat manifested as fullness and tightness in the epigastrium without pain or with slight pain, poor appetite, retching or vomiting, borborygmus, diarrhea, thin yellow and greasy tongue coat, a wiry, rapid pulse.

■ Cautions and Contraindications
It is contraindicated in cases of retching and nausea due to stomach Yin deficiency.

■ Modern Applications
Acute or chronic gastroenteritis, peptic ulcer, indigestion, gastrointestinal neurosis, morning sickness, etc.

Bao He Wan-Preserving Harmony Pill

Citrus and Crataegus Formula
保和丸

■ **Ingredients**

Shan Zha	Crataegus Fruit	180g
Shen Qu	Medicated Leaven	60g
Lai Fu Zi	Radish seed	30g
Ban Xia	Pinellia Tuber	90g
Fu Ling	Hoelen/Poria	90g
Chen Pi	Tangerine Peel	30g
Lian Qiao	Forsythia Fruit	30g

■ **Preparation**

Use as prepared form or decoction with properly reduced dosage.

■ **Pertaining Category**

Food Stagnation Relieving

■ **Functions**

Promotes digestion, removes stagnant food and dampness.
Harmonizes the stomach.

■ **Indications**

Mild food stagnation manifested as a fullness and stuffiness
sensation in the epigastrium, abdominal distention or pain,
belching with foul odor, sour regurgitation, nausea, vomiting, loss
of appetite, or diarrhea, white or yellow greasy tongue coat, a
slippery pulse.

■ **Cautions and Contraindications**

Use with caution for patients with spleen and stomach deficiency.

■ **Modern Applications**

Acute or chronic gastroenteritis, indigestion, etc.

Bei Mu Gua Lou San-Fritillaria and Trichosanthes Fruit Powder
Powder of Fritillary Bulb and Snakegourd Fruit
贝 母 瓜 蒌 散

■ **Ingredients**

Chuan Bei Mu	Tendrilled Fritillary	5g
Gua Lou	Trichosanthes Fruit	3g
Tian Hua Fen	Trichosanthes Root	2.5g
Fu Ling	Hoelen/Poria	2.5g
Chen Pi	Tangerine Peel	2.5g
Jie Geng	Platycodon	2.5g

■ **Preparation**

Use as decoction or prepared form.

■ **Pertaining Category**

Dryness Moistening and Phlegm Resolving

■ **Functions**

Moistens the lungs, clears heat. Regulates Qi, resolves phlegm.

■ **Indications**

Dry phlegm in the lungs with slight injury to Yin manifested as cough with sticky sputum that is hard to expectorate, dry throat, difficulty in breathing, red and dry tongue with scanty coat, a thin, rapid pulse.

■ **Cautions and Contraindications**

It is inappropriate to use this formula for patients with unproductive cough, dry throat, malar flush, and night sweats due to Yin deficiency with deficient fire.

■ **Modern Applications**

Chronic bronchitis, trachitis, pulmonary emphysema, aphonia, etc.

Bei Xie Fen Qing Yin I-Hypoglauca Yam Beverage to Separate the Clear from Turbid

Tokoro Combination
草解分清饮

■ Ingredients

Bei Xie	Hypoglauca Yam	10g
Yi Zhi Ren	Alpinia	10g
Wu Yao	Lindera Root	10g
Shi Chang Pu	Sweetflag Rhizome	10g
Fu Ling	Hoelen/Poria	9g
Gan Cao	Licorice	6g

■ Preparation
Use as decoction or prepared form.

■ Pertaining Category
Yang Warming and Dampness Transforming

■ Functions
Warms the lower burner, drains dampness. Purifies the turbidity.

■ Indications
Damp-cold in the lower burner with kidney Qi and Yang deficiency manifested as frequent, greasy, and cloudy urine, or milky like rice water, soreness of lower back, pale tongue with white coat, a deep, slow, and weak pulse.

■ Cautions and Contraindications
It is contraindicated in cases of the kidney Yin deficiency or milky urine due to damp-heat in the lower burner.

■ Modern Applications
Chronic prostatitis, gonorrhea, chronic pyelonephritis, nephronic syndrome, chronic pelvic inflammatory disease, trichomoniasis, etc. *This formula is from "Dan Xi Xin Fa"(Teachings of Dan Xi).*

Bei Xie Fen Qing Yin II-Hypoglauca Yam Beverage to Separate the Clear from Turbid

Tokoro Combination

萆 解 分 清 饮

■ **Ingredients**

Bei Xie	*Hypoglauca Yam*	10g
Huang Bai	*Phellodendron*	3g
Shi Chang Pu	*Sweetflag Rhizome*	3g
Fu Ling	*Hoelen/Poria*	5g
Bai Zhu	*White Atractylodes*	5g
Lian Zi Xin	*Lotus Seed*	4g
Dan Shen	*Salvia Root*	7g
Che Qian Zi	*Plantago Seed*	7g

■ **Preparation**

Use as decoction or prepared form. Che Qian Zi should be wrapped in gauze when making decoction.

■ **Pertaining Category**

Damp-heat Clearing

■ **Functions**

Clears heat, drains dampness. Purifies the turbidity.

■ **Indications**

Turbid damp-heat in the lower burner manifested as painful and difficult urination with cloudy urine, or dripping cloudy urine, red tongue with yellow greasy coat, a wiry, slippery, and rapid pulse.

■ **Cautions and Contraindications**

None noted.

■ **Modern Applications**

Prostatitis, gonorrhea, acute or chronic pelvic inflammation, trichomoniasis, etc.

This formula is from "Yi Xue Xin Wu" (Medical Revelation).

Bei Xie Shen Shi Tang-Hypoglauca Yam Dampness Draining Decoction

Hypoglauca Yam and Coix Combination

草 解 渗 湿 汤

■ Ingredients

Bei Xie	Hypoglauca Yam	9g
Yi Yi Ren	Coix Seed	15g
Huang Bai	Phellodendron Bark	9g
Fu Ling	Hoelen/Poria	12g
Mu Dan Pi	Moutan Bark	9g
Ze Xie	Alisma	9g
Tong Cao	Rice Paper Pith	6g
Hua Shi	Talcum	15g

■ Preparation
Use as decoction or prepared form.

■ Pertaining Category
Additional Formulas for Ob-Gyn Disorders

■ Functions
Clears damp-heat, relieves toxicity. Kills parasites, stops itching.

■ Indications
Downward flowing of damp-heat in the liver channel manifested as vaginal itching or pain with constant irritation, excessive yellow, foamy, and fishy-smelling vaginal discharge, restlessness, insomnia, a bitter taste in the mouth with a sticky feeling, a fullness and discomfort sensation in the chest, reduced appetite, red tongue with yellow greasy coat, a wiry, rapid pulse.

■ Cautions and Contraindications
Use with caution for patients with deficient spleen and stomach. Do not use for long term.

■ Modern Applications
Leukorrhea, trichomonas vaginalis, etc.

For best result, add Cang Zhu(Atractylodes)9g, Ku Shen(Bitter Ginseng Root)9g, Bai Xian Pi(Dittany)9g.

Bu Fei E Jiao Tang-Tonify the Lungs Decoction with Donkey-hide Gelatin
Donkey-hide Gelatin and Arctium Combination
补 肺 阿 胶 汤

■ **Ingredients**

E Jiao	*Equus/Gelatin*	45g
Niu Bang Zi	*Arctium*	7.5g
Xing Ren	*Apricot Seed*	6g
Ma Dou Ling	*Aristolochia*	15g
Geng Mi	*Oryza*	30g
Zhi Gan Cao	*Baked Licorice*	7.5g

■ **Preparation**
Use as decoction. E Jiao should be dissolved in boiling water, then added into the strained decoction.

■ **Pertaining Category**
Yin Tonifying

■ **Functions**
Nourishes the lung Yin, stops coughing and bleeding.

■ **Indications**
Deficiency of the lung Yin with lung heat manifested as dry cough with scanty sputum, or blood tinged sputum, or coughing of blood, difficulty in breathing, dry throat, slight thirst, red tongue with scanty coat, a superficial, thin, and rapid pulse.

■ **Cautions and Contraindications**
Do not use overdose and for long term.

■ **Modern Applications**
Chronic bronchitis, pneumonia, pulmonary tuberculosis, etc.

Bu Fei Tang-Tonify the Lungs Decoction
Astragalus and Aster Combination
补 肺 汤

■ **Ingredients**

Huang Qi	Astragalus	12-20g
Shu Di Huang	Cooked Rehmannia	12-20g
Ren Shen	Ginseng	6-9g
Zi Wan	Purple Aster Root	6-9g
Sang Bai Pi	Morus Rootbark	9-12g
Wu Wei Zi	Schisandra	6-9g

■ **Preparation**
Use as decoction or prepared form.

■ **Pertaining Category**
Qi Tonigying

■ **Functions**
Tonifies the lung Qi, strengthens defensive Qi, nourishes lung Yin, stops coughing.

■ **Indications**
Lung Qi deficiency manifested as cough with thin, clear, and scant sputum, shortness of breath, low voice, fatigue, pale complexion, spontaneous sweating, aversion to cold, slight thirst, pale and dry tongue with thin white coat, a weak, frail pulse.

■ **Cautions and Contraindications**
None noted.

■ **Modern Applications**
Chronic bronchitis, chronic bronchial asthma, pulmonary emphysema, etc.

Bu Gan Tang-Tonify the Liver Decoction
补肝汤

■ **Ingredients**

Shu Di Huang	Cooked Rehmannia	9-20g
Dang Gui	Chinese Angelica	9-12g
Bai Shao Yao	White Peony	9-15g
Chuan Xiong	Ligusticum	6-9g
Mu Gua	Chaenomeles Fruit	6-9g
Suan Zao Ren	Zizyphus	6-9g
Mai Men Dong	Ophiopogon	6-9g
Zhi Gan Cao	Baked Licorice	3-6g

■ **Preparation**
Use as decoction or prepared form.

■ **Pertaining Category**
Blood Tonifying

■ **Functions**
Tonifies the liver blood, nourishes the liver Yin. Harmonizes blood circulation.

■ **Indications**
Liver blood and Yin deficiency manifested as dizziness, blurred vision, headache, dry eyes, numbness of limbs or muscle twitches, or amenorrhea, pale or red dry tongue with thin white or thin yellow coat, a wiry, thin, or slight rapid pulse.

■ Cautions and Contraindications
Use with caution for patients with diarrhea due to spleen deficiency or excessive menstrual bleeding.

■ Modern Applications
Anemia, postpartum anemia, irregular menstruation, etc.

Bu Huan Jin Zheng Qi San-Qi Rectifying Powder Worth More Than Gold
Pinellia, Atractylodes, and Agastache Formula
不 换 金 正 气 散

■ Ingredients

Ban Xia	*Pinellia Tuber*	6-9g
Cang Zhu	*Atractylodes*	6-9g
Huo Xiang	*Agstache*	6-9g
Chen Pi	*Tangerine Peel*	6-9g
Hou Po	*Magnolia Bark*	6-9g
Gan Cao	*Licorice*	3-6g
Sheng Jiang	*Fresh Ginger*	3slices
Da Zao	*Jujube*	2pcs

■ Preparation
Use as prepared form or decoction.

■ Pertaining Category
Dampness Drying and Stomach Harmonizing

■ Functions
Moves Qi, transforms turbid dampness. Harmonizes the stomach, descends the rebellious Qi, stops vomiting.

■ Indications
External wind-cold with turbid dampness attacking stomach and intestines manifested as chills, fever, vomiting, diarrhea, fullness of epigastrium, abdominal distention and pain, white greasy tongue coat, a superficial, slippery pulse.

■ Cautions and Contraindications
It is contraindicated in cases of red tongue with scanty coat due to Yin deficiency.

■ Modern Applications
Cholera, acute gastroenteritis, colitis, hepatitis, etc.

Bu Yang Huan Wu Tang-Tonify Yang to Restore Five Decoction
Astragalus and Peony Combination
补 阳 还 五 汤

■ Ingredients

Sheng Huang Qi	Astragalus	120g
Dang Gui	Chinese Angelica	6g
Chuan Xiong	Ligusticum	3g
Chi Shao Yao	Red Peony	6g
Tao Ren	Peach Kernel	3g
Hong Hua	Safflower	3g
Di Long	Earthworm	3g

■ Preparation
Use as decoction or prepared form.

■ Pertaining Category
Blood Invigorating

■ Functions

Tonifies Qi, promotes blood circulation, removes blood stasis, unblocks the channels.

■ Indications

Qi deficiency with blood stasis obstructing the channels manifested as hemiplegia, deviation of the mouth and eye, salivation, slurred speech, atrophy and disability of lower limbs, frequent urination or incontinence, purple tongue with white coat, a slow, weak pulse.

■ Cautions and Contraindications

This formula should be used when patient has regained clear consciousness and normal body temperature, cerebral hemorrhage has arrested. It is contraindicated in cases of stirring up of liver wind, phlegm obstructing in the channels, Yin deficiency, and heat in the blood as well as during pregnancy.

■ Modern Applications

Sequelae of cerebrovascular accident, sequelae of poliomyelitis, paralysis of extremity due to other diseases or trauma, etc.

The dosage of Astragalus may begin with 30-60g and increased gradually to 120g. The formula should be taken for a certain period of time after recovery to prevent relapse.

Bu Zhong Yi Qi Tang-Reinforce the Middle Burner and Tonify Qi Decoction
Ginseng and Astragalus Combination
补中益气汤

■ Ingredients

Ren Shen	Ginseng	10g
Huang Qi	Astragalus	15g
Bai Zhu	White Atractylodes	10g
Dang Gui	Chinese Angelica	10g
Chen Pi	Tangerine Peel	6g
Chai Hu	Bupleurum	3g
Sheng Ma	Cimicufuga	3g
Zhi Gan Cao	Baked Licorice	5g

■ Preparation
Use as decoction or prepared form.

■ Pertaining Category
Qi Tonifying

■ Functions
Tonifies the spleen and stomach Qi, lifts Yang Qi.

■ Indications
Deficiency and sinking of the spleen and stomach Qi manifested as shortness of breath, weak voice, lassitude, tastelessness, lack of appetite, prolapse of visceras, prolonged diarrhea and dysentery, chronic uterine bleeding, or persistent lower grade fever, headache, dizziness, spontaneous sweating, aversion to cold, thirst with a desire to drink warm fluids, pale tongue with white coat, a weak, feeble pulse.

■ Cautions and Contraindications
It is contraindicated in cases of lower grade fever due to Yin deficiency.

■ Modern Applications
Gastroptosis, prolapse of the rectum and uterus, lower blood pressure, myasthenia gravis, uterine bleeding, chronic bleeding, chronic gastroenteritis, post-surgical recovery, etc.

Cang Er Zi San-Xanthium Powder
Xanthium Formula
苍耳子散

■ **Ingredients**

Cang Er Zi	*Xanthium fruit*	6-9g
Xin Yi	*Magnolia Flower*	3-6g
Bai Zhi	*Angelica Root*	6-9g
Bo He	*Peppermint*	3-6g

■ **Preparation**
Use as prepared form or decoction.

■ **Pertaining Category**
External Wind Expelling

■ **Functions**
Expels wind, relieves pain. Opens the nasal orifices.

■ **Indications**
Wind invasion affecting the nasal cavity manifested as nasal congestion with thick nasal discharge, frontal headache, yellow tongue coat, a superficial, rapid pulse.

■ **Cautions and Contraindications**
None noted.

■ **Modern Applications**
Acute, chronic, and allergic rhinitis, acute or chronic sinusitis, etc.

Chai Ge Jie Ji Tang-Bupleurum and Pueraria Release Muscle Layer Decoction
Bupleurum and Pueraria Combination
柴葛解肌汤

■ Ingredients

Chai Hu	Bupleurum	6g
Ge Gen	Pueraria	9g
Huang Qin	Scute	6g
Qiang Huo	Notopterygium	3g
Bai Zhi	Angelica Root	3g
Bai Shao Yao	White Peony	6g
Shi Gao	Gypsum	5g
Jie Geng	Platycodon	3g
Gan Cao	Licorice	3g
Sheng Jiang	Fresh Ginger	3slices
Da Zao	Jujube	2pcs

■ Preparation
Use as decoction or prepared form. Do not cook for more than 20 minutes.

■ Pertaining Category
Pungent Cool Exterior Relieving

■ Functions
Expels wind-cold or wind-heat, releases pathogen from muscle layer, relieves pain. Clears internal heat.

■ Indications
Exterior wind-cold or wind-heat invasion with interior heat (both Wei and Qi level affection) manifested as slight aversion to cold, high fever, headache, body aches, soreness and pain in the limbs, orbital and eye pain, dry nose, restlessness, insomnia, red tongue with thin yellow coat, a superficial, slight full, and rapid pulse.

■ Cautions and Contraindications

It is contraindicated in cases of only exterior wind-cold without heat or only internal heat with constipation and abdominal pain. It is unnecessary to use this formula for mild exterior wind-heat invasion.

■ Modern Applications

Common cold, influenza, acute bronchitis, trigeminal neuralgia, toothache, headaches, etc.

This formula is from "Shang Han Liu Shu "(Six Texts on Cold-induced Disorders).

Chai Hu Da Yuan Yin-Bupleurum Beverage to Reach the Primary Membrane
Bupleurum and Scute Combination
柴 胡 达 原 饮

■ Ingredients

Chai Hu	Bupleurum	5g
Zhi Ke	Bitter Orange	5g
Hou Po	Magnolia Bark	5g
Qing Pi	Green Citrus Peel	5g
Huang Qin	Scute	5g
Jie Geng	Platycodon	3g
Cao Guo	Tsaoko	2g
Bing Lang	Areca	6g
He Ye Geng	Nelumbo	10-15g
Zhi Gan Cao	Baked Licorice	2g

■ Preparation

Use as decoction.

■ Pertaining Category

Shaoyang Harmonizing (Mediating)

■ **Functions**

Transforms phlegm and dampness, dispels pathogen at the level of the membrane source (between exterior and interior), harmonizes Shaoyang.

■ **Indications**

Phlegm-dampness retention complicated with Shaoyang disorder caused by invasion of dampness obstructing the membrane source affecting both exterior and interior manifested as fullness in the chest, diaphragm, and epigastrium, irritability, dizziness, stickiness in the mouth, cough with sputum that is difficult to expectorate, malaria attack with alternate chills and fever, thick pasty tongue coat, a wiry, slippery pulse.

■ **Cautions and Contraindications**

None noted.

■ **Modern Applications**

Malarial disorders, respiratory or digestive disorders, etc.

Chai Hu Gui Zhi Tang-Bupleurum and Cinnamon Twig Decoction
Bupleurum and Cinnamon Combination
柴 胡 桂 枝 汤

■ **Ingredients**

Chai Hu	Bupleurum	9g
Gui Zhi	Cinnamon Twig	6g
Ren Shen	Ginseng	6g
Ban Xia	Pinellia Tuber	6g
Huang Qin	Scute	6g
Bai Shao Yao	White Peony	6g
Sheng Jiang	Fresh Ginger	6g
Da Zao	Jujube	4pcs
Gan Cao	Licorice	3g

■ **Preparation**

Use as decoction or prepared form.

■ **Pertaining Category**

Relieving Both Exterior and Interior

■ **Functions**

Expels external pathogen, releases the exterior and muscle layer. Harmonizes the Shaoyang, benefits the joints.

■ **Indications**

Shaoyang syndrome with unreleased exterior condition manifested as mild chills, fever, or alternate chills and fever, nausea, joint pain, or epigastric fullness and pain due to disharmony between liver and spleen, thin white tongue coat, a wiry pulse.

■ **Cautions and Contraindications**

This formula is rather warm than cool, it should not be used for excessive heat conditions.

■ **Modern Applications**

Common cold with digestive disorder, influenza, gastritis, jaundice, cholecystitis, chronic appendicitis, intercostal neuralgia, mild arthritis, etc.

This formula is a combination of Xiao Chai Hu Tang and Gui Zhi Tang with both reduced dosages.

Chai Hu Jia Long Gu Mu Li Tang- Bupleurum plus Dragon Bone and Oyster Shell Decoction
Bupleurum and Dragon Bone Combination
柴 胡 加 龙 骨 牡 蛎 汤

Ingredients

Chai Hu	Bupleurum	9-12g
Huang Qin	Scute	4.5-6g
Ren Shen	Ginseng	4.5-6g
Gui Zhi	Cinnamon Twig	4.5g
Ban Xia	Pinellia Tuber	6-9g
Fu Ling	Hoelen/Poria	6g
Da Huang	Rhubarb	6g
Long Gu	Drangon Bone	6g
Mu Li	Oyster Shell	6g
Sheng Jiang	Fresh Ginger	3-6g
Da Zao	Jujube	3-6pcs
Qian Dan	Minium	1-4g

■ Preparation
Use as decoction or prepared form.

■ Pertaining Category
Spirit Calming with Heavy Sedative Herbs

■ Functions
Harmonizes the Shaoyang channel, purges heat, calms spirit.

■ Indications
Evil heat invading from Taiyang into Shaoyang and Yangming with disturbance of spirit and Qi deficiency manifested as irritability, a fullness sensation in the chest, difficult urination, constipation, delirious speech, general heaviness with difficulty in rotating the trunk, red tongue with greasy coat, a wiry, rapid pulse.

■ Cautions and Contraindications
Use with caution during pregnancy. Qian Dan (Minium) is toxic; it should be substituted by Dai Zhe Shi (Hematite) with dosage of 10-15g.

■ Modern Applications
Neurosis, schizophrenia, hysteria, epilepsy, hyperthyroidism, menopausal syndrome, hypertension, etc.

Chai Hu Shu Gan San-Bupleurum Powder to Disperse Liver Qi

Bupleurum and Cyperus Combination

柴 胡 疏 肝 散

■ Ingredients

Chai Hu	Bupleurum	6g
Chuan Xiong	Ligusticum	4.5g
Xiang Fu	Cyperus	4.5g
Chen Pi	Tangerine Peel	6g
Zhi Ke	Bitter Orange	4.5g
Bai Shao Yao	White Peony	4.5g
Zhi Gan Cao	Baked Licorice	1.5g

■ Preparation
Use as decoction or prepared form.

■ Pertaining Category
Regulating the Liver and Spleen (Mediating)

■ Functions
Disperses liver Qi, harmonizes blood, relieves pain.

■ Indications
Constraint of the liver Qi with mild blood stagnation manifested as mental depression, hypochondriac distention or pain, a fullness sensation in the chest, belching, painful menstruation, breast distention, or alternate chills and fever, thin white tongue coat, a wiry pulse.

■ Cautions and Contraindications
None noted.

■ Modern Applications
Dysmenorrhea, premenstrual syndrome, irregular menstruation, fibrocystic breasts, gastritis, peptic ulcer, hepatitis, cholecystitis, pancreatitis, intercostal neuralgia, etc.

Chuan Xiong Cha Tiao San-Ligusticum Green Tea Mixture
Cnidium and Tea Formula
川芎茶调散

■ **Ingredients**

Chuan Xiong	Ligusticum	120g
Jing Jie	Schizonepeta	120g
Bai Zhi	Angelica Root	60g
Qiang Huo	Notopterygium	60g
Xi Xin	Asarum	30g
Fang Feng	Siler	45g
Bo He	Peppermint	240g
Gan Cao	Licorice	60g

■ **Preparation**

Use as prepared form and take with green tea, or use as decoction with properly reduced dosage.

■ **Pertaining Category**

External Wind Expelling

■ **Functions**

Expels wind-cold, relieves pain.

■ **Indications**

External wind-cold invading and affecting the head manifested as recurrent headache (frontal, temporal, occipital, vertex, or migraine), aversion to cold, fever, blurred vision, vertigo, stuffy nose, thin white tongue coat, a superficial, tight pulse.

■ Cautions and Contraindications
It is contraindicated in cases of headache due to deficiency of Qi and blood, liver wind, or liver Yang raising. Do not use overdose and for long term.

■ Modern Applications
Migraine, headache, common cold, headache due to rhinitis, nervous headache, trigeminal neuralgia, etc.

Ci Zhu Wan-Magnetite and Cinnabar Pill
Magnetite and Cinnabar Combination
磁朱丸

■ Ingredients

Ci Shi	Magnetite	60g
Zhu Sha	Cinnabar	30g
Shen Qu	Medicated Leaven	120g

■ Preparation
Use as prepared form.

■ Pertaining Category
Spirit Calming with Heavy Sedative Herbs

■ Functions
Sedates the heart fire, calms spirit. Suppresses Yang, benefits Yin and essence, improves hearing and vision.

■ Indications
Disharmony between the kidney water and heart fire manifested as palpitation, insomnia, tinnitus, deafness, blurred vision, dizziness, headache, or seizures, red tongue with thin yellow coat or no coat, thin, rapid or wiry, rapid pulse.

■ Cautions and Contraindications

Do not use overdose and for long term, or during pregnancy. Use with caution for patients with a weak digestive system. It should be modified significantly for visual and hearing problem due to liver and kidney deficiency.

■ Modern Applications

Insomnia, tachycardia, vegetative nerve dysfunction, neurosis, cataract, glaucoma, optic nerve atrophy, epilepsy, tinnitus, or schizophrenia, etc.

Cong Chi Jie Geng Tang-Scallion, Prepared Soybean, and Platycodon Decoction
葱豉桔梗汤

■ Ingredients

Cong Bai	Allium Bulb	3 piece
Jie Geng	Platycodon	3-4.5g
Zhi Zi	Gardenia Fruit	6-9g
Dan Dou Chi	Prepared Soybean	9-15g
Bo He	Peppermint	3-4.5g
Lian Qiao	Forsythia Fruit	4.5-6g
Dan Zhu Ye	Bland Bamboo Leaf	3g
Gan Cao	Licorice	2g

■ Preparation

Use as decoction or prepared form. Do not cook for more than 20 minutes. Bo He should be added 5 minutes near the end of cooking.

■ Pertaining Category

Pungent Cool Exterior Relieving

■ Functions

Expels wind-heat, relieves the exterior. Clears the lung heat.

■ Indications

Exterior wind-heat invasion with lung heat manifested as headache, fever, mild aversion to wind-cold, cough, sore throat, thirst, red tip tongue with thin white coat, a superficial, rapid pulse.

■ Cautions and Contraindications

None noted.

■ Modern Applications

Common cold, laryngopharyngitis, bronchitis, etc.

Da Bu Yin Wan-Great Tonify Yin Pill
Pills for Replenishing the Yin
大 补 阴 丸

■ Ingredients

Shu Di Huang	Cooked Rehmannia	180g
Zhi Mu	Anemarrhena	120g
Huang Bai	Phellodendron	120g
Gui Ban	Tortoise Plastron	180g
Zhu Ji Sui	Bone Marrow of Pig	Proper Amount

■ Preparation

Use as prepared form.

■ Pertaining Category

Yin Tonifying

■ Functions

Nourishes the kidney Yin, reduces deficient fire.

■ Indications

Deficiency of the kidney Yin with deficient fire flaring up manifested as tidal fever or steaming bone fever, night sweats, nocturnal emission, coughing of blood, irritability, easy to get angry, painful, feverish, and weakness of the knees and feet, red tongue with scanty coat, a rapid, forceful pulse in the rear position.

■ Cautions and Contraindications

It is contraindicated in cases of poor appetite and diarrhea due to deficiency of the spleen and stomach or excess heat patterns.

■ Modern Applications

Diabetes, chronic nephritis, tinnitus, hyperthyroidism, prostatitis, pulmonary, renal, or bone tuberculosis, etc.

Da Bu Yuan Jian-Great Tonify the Primary Brew
Ginseng and Rehmannia Combination
大 补 元 煎

■ Ingredients

Ren Shen	Ginseng	6g
Shu Di Huang	Cooked Rehmannia	9-15g
Shan Yao	Dioscorea	6g
Shan Zhu Yu	Dogwood Fruit	3-6g
Gou Qi Zi	Lycium Fruit	6g
Dang Gui	Chinese Angelica	6g
Du Zhong	Eucommia	6g
Zhi Gan Cao	Baked Licorice	3g

■ Preparation

Use as decoction or prepared form.

■ Pertaining Category

Yin Tonifying

■ Functions

Nourishes the kidney Yin, strengthens the kidney and spleen Qi, enriches blood.

■ Indications

Kidney Yin and Qi deficiency with spleen Qi and blood deficiency manifested as soreness and weakness of lower back, tinnitus and loss of hearing, uterine bleeding or prolapse, frequent urination, red or pale tongue, a thin, weak pulse.

■ Cautions and Contraindications

None noted.

■ Modern Applications

Uterine bleeding, uterine prolapse, chronic nephritis, etc.

Da Chai Hu Tang-Major Bupleurum Decoction
Major Bupleurum Combination
大 柴 胡 汤

■ Ingredients

Chai Hu	Bupleurum	15g
Huang Qin	Scute	9g
Bai Shao Yao	White Peony	9g
Ban Xia	Pinellia Tuber	9g
Zhi Shi	Immature Citrus	9g
Da Huang	Rhubarb	6g
Sheng Jiang	Fresh Ginger	15g
Da Zao	Jujube	5pcs

■ Preparation

Use as decoction or prepared form.

■ **Pertaining Category**
Relieving Both Exterior and Interior

■ **Functions**
Harmonizes the Shaoyang channel. Purges the interior accumulated heat.

■ **Indications**
Shaoyang disorders with heat accumulating in the Yangming Fu organ manifested as alternate chills and fever, fullness and discomfort in the chest and hypochondrium, nausea, vomiting, mental depression or irritability, epigastric fullness, pain, or rigidity, constipation or hesitant bowel movement, or foul diarrhea with a burning sensation in the anus, light red tongue with yellow coat, a wiry, rapid pulse.

■ **Cautions and Contraindications**
It is contraindicated in cases of exterior patterns or Shaoyang disorders without internal heat.

■ **Modern Applications**
Acute cholecystitis, cholelithiasis, acute pancreatitis, simple intestinal obstruction, peritonitis, hepatitis, gastroenteritis, dysentery pleurisy, malaria, etc.

Da Cheng Qi Tang-Major Decoction for Purging Down Digestive Qi
Major Rhubarb Combination
大承气汤

■ **Ingredients**

Da Huang	*Rhubarb*	12g
Mang Xiao	*Mirabilitum*	9g
Zhi Shi	*Immature Citrus*	12g
Hou Po	*Magnolia Bark*	15g

■ **Preparation**

Use as decoction or prepared form. Da Huang (Rhubarb) should be added at last 3-5 minutes when making decoction; Mang Xiao (Mirabilitum) should be infused in the decoction that made from other ingredients.

■ **Pertaining Category**

Purging Downward with Cold Nature

■ **Functions**

Purges heat, moves Qi downward, promotes bowel movement.

■ **Indications**

Excessive heat accumulating in the Yangming Fu organ manifested as constipation or watery dysentery with odorous stools, frequent passing gas, abdominal fullness and pain which is aggravated by pressure, or abdominal palpable hard mass, tidal fever and sweating of hands and feet, delirium, or mania, dry mouth and tongue with yellow, black, dry coat, a deep, forceful or slippery, forceful pulse; or syncope and convulsion due to excess heat.

■ **Cautions and Contraindications**

It is contraindicated in cases of weak constitution, exterior patterns, and women during pregnancy. It should be discontinued immediately after the bowel has moved.

■ **Modern Applications**

Acute appendicitis, acute cholecystitis, acute pancreatitis, acute uncomplicated intestinal obstruction, syncope, seizures, roundworm in the bile duct, early stage of dysentery, food poisoning, etc.

Da Ding Feng Zhu-Major Arrest Wind Pearl
The Big Pearl for Endogenous Wind
大 定 风 珠

Ingredients

Bai Shao Yao	*White Peony*	18g
E Jiao	*Equus/Gelatin*	9g
Gui Ban	*Tortoise Plastron*	12g
Sheng Di Huang	*Dried Rehmannia*	18g
Huo Ma Ren	*Hemp Seed*	6g
Wu Wei Zi	*Schisandra*	6g
Mu Li	*Oyster Shell*	12g
Mai Men Dong	*Ophiopogon*	18g
Ji Zi Huang	*Egg Yolk*	2pcs
Bie Jia	*Tortoise Shell*	12g
Zhi Gan Cao	*Baked Licorice*	12g

Preparation

Use as decoction. E Jiao should be dissolved separately in boiling water and added into strained decoction. Bie Jia, Mu Li, and Gui Ban should be crushed and cooked 45 minutes prior to the other herbs. Egg Yolks are boiled hard and mixed into the decoction.

Pertaining Category

Internal Wind Extinguishing

Functions

Nourishes Yin, suppresses the liver Yang, extinguishes wind.

Indications

Endogenous wind due to severe Yin deficiency manifested as twitches and spasms of muscles, trembling of hands, chronic convulsion, listlessness, fatigue, or tendency to go into prostration, dark red tongue with scanty coat, a weak, frail pulse.

Cautions and Contraindications

It is contraindicated in cases of Yin deficiency with excess pathogenic heat. Use with extreme caution during pregnancy.

Modern Applications

Encephalitis, meningitis, Parkinson's disease, chronic convulsion, hepatic coma, etc.

Da Huang Fu Zi Tang-Rhubarb and Prepared Aconite Decoction
Rhubarb and Aconite Combination
大 黄 附 子 汤

■ **Ingredients**

Da Huang	Rhubarb	9g
Pao Fu Zi	Prepared Aconite	9g
Xi Xin	Asarum	3g

■ **Preparation**
Use as decoction or prepared form.

■ **Pertaining Category**
Purging Downward with Warm Nature

■ **Functions**
Warms Yang, dispels cold. Purges stagnation to relieve constipation, stops pain.

■ **Indications**
Interior cold accumulation manifested as constipation, abdominal pain, hypochondriac pain, extreme cold limbs, white greasy tongue coat, a wiry, tense pulse.

■ **Cautions and Contraindications**
It is contraindicated for pregnant woman. The dosage of Da Huang (Rhubarb) should not be bigger than Fu Zi (Prepared Aconite).

■ **Modern Applications**
Chronic dysentery, ulcerative colitis, uncomplicated appendicitis, intestinal obstruction without complication, hernia, etc.
If the patient dose not respond to the treatment and still remains constipated with cold limbs, these indicate critical condition, the patient needs an emergent care.

Da Huang Mu Dan Tang-Rhubarb and Moutan Decoction
Rhubarb and Moutan Combination
大黄牡丹汤

■ **Ingredients**

Da Huang	Rhubarb	12-18g
Mu Dan Pi	Moutan Bark	9g
Tao Ren	Peach Kernel	12g
Dong Gua Ren	Benincasa	30g
Mang Xiao	Mirabilite	9g

■ **Preparation**

Use as decoction or prepared form. Da Huang should be added 4-5 minutes near the end of making decoction; Mang Xiao should be infused into strained decoction.

■ **Pertaining Category**

Treating Internal Abscess

■ **Functions**

Purges heat, breaks up blood stasis, reduces swelling, disperses pathogenic accumulation.

■ **Indications**

Intestinal abscess from toxic damp-heat and stagnant blood in the intestines manifested as tenderness and pain in the right lower abdomen with limitation of extending the right leg, the pain is aggravated by pressure, fever, chills followed by sweating, red tongue with thin yellow greasy coat, a slippery, rapid pulse.

■ **Cautions and Contraindications**

It is contraindicated during pregnancy. Use with extreme caution for elderly and patients with weak constitution.

■ **Modern Applications**

Early stage of acute appendicitis without complication, pelvic inflammatory disease, acute annexitis, mesenteric lymphadenitis, lochioschesis, etc.

Da Jian Zhong Tang-Major Strengthen the Middle Burner Decoction
Major Zanthoxylum Combination
大 建 中 汤

■ **Ingredients**

Hua Jiao	*Zanthoxylum*	3-9g
Gan Jiang	*Dried Ginger*	12g
Ren Shen	*Ginseng*	6g
Yi Tang	*Maltose*	18-30g

■ **Preparation**

Use as decoction or prepared form.

■ **Pertaining Category**

Middle Burner Warming and Cold Dispelling

■ **Functions**

Warms and tonifies the middle burner, dispels cold. Descends the rebellious stomach Qi, relieves spasmodic abdominal pain.

■ Indications

Spleen Yang deficiency with severe cold stagnation manifested as severe epigastric and abdominal cramping pain to the point that patient can be barely touched, a strong cold sensation in the epigastric region, borborygmus, vomiting with inability to eat, or vomiting of round worms, pale or purple tongue with white greasy coat, a wiry, slow, deep, or thin pulse.

■ Cautions and Contraindications

It is contraindicated in cases of interior damp-heat, or Yin and blood deficiency.

■ Modern Applications

Peptic ulcer, biliary ascariasis, pancreatitis, gastric and intestinal spasms, uncomplicated intestinal obstruction, etc.

This formula has stronger effects of tonifying deficiency and dispelling cold than Xiao Jian Zhong Tang (Minor Strengthen the Middle Burner Decoction).

Da Qin Jiao Tang-Large Leaf Gentiana Root Decoction
Major Gentiana Qin Jiao Decoction
大秦芄汤

■ Ingredients

Qin Jiao	Big Leaf Gentiana	90g
Chuan Xiong	Ligusticum	60g
Dang Gui	Chinese Angelica	60g
Bai Shao Yao	White Peony	60g
Xi Xin	Asarum	15g
Qiang Huo	Notopterygium	30g
Du Huo	Tuhuo	60g
Fang Feng	Siler	30g
Huang Qin	Scute	30g
Shi Gao	Gypsum	60g
Bai Zhu	White Atractylodes	30g
Bai Zhi	Angelica Root	30g
Sheng Di Huang	Dried Rehmannia	30g
Shu Di Huang	Cooked Rehmannia	30g
Fu Ling	Hoelen/Poria	30g
Gan Cao	Licorice	60g

■ Preparation
Use as prepared form or decoction with properly reduced dosage.

■ Pertaining Category
External Wind Expelling

■ Functions
Expels wind-dampness, Clears heat. Nourishes blood, promotes blood circulation.

■ Indications

External wind-dampness attacking channels and turning to heat with Qi and blood deficiency manifested as sudden deviation of mouth and eyes, stiffness of tongue with slurred speech, rigidity of the extremities, failure to move the hands and feet, or spasms of muscles, numbness of the limbs and aching joints, or accompanied by chills and fever, a white or yellow tongue coat, a superficial and tight, or wiry, rapid pulse.

Cautions and Contraindications

It is contraindicated for patients with endogenous wind. Do not use overdose and for long term.

Modern Applications

Arthritis, sequelae of poliomyelitis, facial paralysis, etc.

Da Qing Long Tang-Major Blue-green Dragon Decoction
Major Blue Dragon Combination
大 青 龙 汤

Ingredients

Ma Huang	Ephedra	12g
Gui Zhi	Cinnamon Twig	6g
Zhi Gan Cao	Baked Licorice	6g
Xing Ren	Apricot Seed	6g
Shi Gao	Gypsum	12g
Sheng Jiang	Fresh Ginger	9g
Da Zao	Jujube	3pcs

Preparation

Use as decoction or prepared form.

Pertaining Category

Pungent Warm Exterior Relieving

Functions

Promotes sweat, releases the exterior. Clears internal heat, relieves irritability.

Indications

Exterior wind-cold with interior heat manifested as severe aversion to cold and fever without sweating, irritability, body aches, asthma, thin white or yellow tongue coat, a superficial, tight pulse.

- **Cautions and Contraindications**

It is contraindicated in cases of exterior deficiency with spontaneous sweating and weak constitution. Use with caution for patients with hypertension and heart problems.

- **Modern Applications**

Common cold, influenza, pleurisy with cough, acute bronchitis, pneumonia, etc.

This formula is modified from Ma Huang Tang (Ephedra Decoction).

Da Xian Xiong Tang-Major Sinking into the Chest Decoction
Rhubarb and Kansui Combination
大陷胸汤

- **Ingredients**

Da Huang	Rhubarb	10g
Mang Xiao	Mirabilitum	10g
Gan Sui	Kansui Spurge Root	1g

- **Preparation**

Use as decoction. Da Huang (Rhubarb) is decocted first, then other two herbs are ground into fine powder and infused in the decoction.

- **Pertaining Category**

Purging Downward with Cold Nature

- **Functions**

Purges heat, eliminates water retention by flushing downward.

■ Indications

Accumulation of heat with phlegm-fluid in the chest and abdomen manifested as fullness, pain from the epigastrium to the lower abdomen, which is aggravated by touching, constipation, mild tidal fever, or shortness of breath, irritability, thirst, dry tongue, a deep, tense, and forceful pulse.

■ Cautions and Contraindications

It is contraindicated for patients with weak constitution or during pregnancy. This formula is drastic and toxic, it should be discontinued immediately after the effect attained.

■ Modern Applications

Inflammatory hydrothorax, ascites, acute edematous pancreatitis, severe intestinal obstruction, peritonitis, cirrhosis, intercostal neuralgia, pulmonary edema, etc.

Dan Shen Yin-Salvia Root Decoction
Salvia Decoction
丹 参 饮

■ Ingredients

Dan Shen	Salvia Root	30g
Sha Ren	Amomum Fruit	5g
Tan Xiang	Santalum	5g

■ Preparation

Use as decoction or prepared form.

■ Pertaining Category

Blood Invigorating

■ Functions

Promotes blood circulation, removes blood stasis. Moves Qi, stops pain.

■ Indications

Stagnation of blood and Qi in the upper and middle burners manifested as intermittent pain in the chest, that may radiate to the upper back and shoulder, a stifling sensation in the chest, shortness of breath, or pain in the epigastrium and abdomen, purple tongue with purplish spots, a wiry, tight, and hesitant pulse.

■ Cautions and Contraindications

It is contraindicated during pregnancy and in cases of excessive menstrual bleeding, bleeding diathesis, or any bleeding disorders, etc.

■ Modern Applications

Angina pectoris, chronic gastritis, pancreatitis, hepatitis, or dysmenorrhea, etc.

Dang Gui Bu Xue Tang-Tang-kuei Tonify Blood Decoction

Tang-kuei and Astragalus Combination

当归补血汤

■ Ingredients

| Huang Qi | *Astragalus* | 30g |
| Dang Gui | *Chinese Angelica* | 6-9g |

■ Preparation

Use as decoction or prepared form.

■ Pertaining Category

Qi and Blood Tonifying

■ Functions

Tonifies Qi, nourishes blood.

■ **Indications**

Qi and blood deficiency with deficient Yang floating to body surface manifested as fever without high body temperature, flushed face, thirst with a desire to drink warm water, or headache and low fever after excessive menstruation or giving birth, fatigue, sallow complexion, or prolonged healing of ulcer, pale tongue with thin coat, a flooding, large, but forceless pulse.

■ **Cautions and Contraindications**

Use with caution in cases of tidal fever due to Yin deficiency.

■ **Modern Applications**

Anemia, allergic purpura, functional uterine bleeding, leukopenia, etc.

Dang Gui Liu Huang Tang-Tang-kuei and Six Yellow Decoction
Chinese Angelica and Six Yellow Ingredients Combination
当归六黄汤

■ **Ingredients**

Dang Gui	Chinese Angelica	9g
Sheng Di Huang	Dried Rehmannia	9g
Shu Di Huang	Cooked Rehmanni	9g
Huang Qin	Scute	9g
Huang Lian	Coptis	9g
Huang Bai	Phellodendron	9g
Huang Qi	Astragalus	18g

■ **Preparation**

Use as decoction or prepared form.

■ **Pertaining Category**

Deficient Heat Clearing

■ **Functions**
Nourishes Yin, drains fire. Consolidates the exterior, stops sweating.

■ **Indications**
Yin deficiency with interior heat manifested as fever, profuse sweating, red face, irritability, dry mouth and lips, constipation, yellow urine, red cracked tongue, a thin, rapid pulse.

■ **Cautions and Contraindications**
Use with caution or in modified form for patients with spleen and stomach deficiency.

■ **Modern Applications**
Tuberculosis, chronic febrile disease, hyperthyroidism, chronic nephritis, neurasthenia, etc.

Dang Gui Long Hui Wan-Tang-kuei, Gentiana, and Aloe Pill
Tang-kuei, Gentiana, and Aloe Formula
当 归 龙 荟 丸

■ **Ingredients**

Dang Gui	*Chinese Angelica*	30g
Long Dan Cao	*Gentiana*	15g
Zhi Zi	*Gardenia Fruit*	30g
Huang Lian	*Coptis*	30g
Huang Bai	*Phellodendron*	30g
Huang Qin	*Scute*	30g
Lu Hui	*Aloe*	15g
Da Huang	*Rhubarb*	15g
Mu Xiang	*Saussurea*	5g
She Xiang	*Musk*	1.5g
Qing Dai	*Indigo*	15g

■ **Preparation**

Grind all ingredients into powder and form into pills with water.

■ **Pertaining Category**

Clearing Heat from Zang-fu Organs

■ **Functions**

Purges the liver and gallbladder excess fire.

■ **Indications**

Excess fire in the liver and gallbladder manifested as headache, vertigo, restlessness, delirium, or mania and convulsion, hypochondriac pain, a bitter taste in the mouth, dry throat, constipation, dark, scanty, and difficult urination, red tongue with yellow coat, a wiry, rapid pulse.

■ **Cautions and Contraindications**

Use with extreme caution for patients with deficiency of the spleen and stomach.

■ **Modern Applications**

Hypertension, acute hepatitis, acute conjunctivitis, cholecystitis, mania, convulsion, acute leukemia, nosebleeding, etc.

Dang Gui Si Ni Tang-Tang Kuei and Four Frigid Limbs Decoction

Tang Kuei and Jujube Combination

当 归 四 逆 汤

■ Ingredients

Dang Gui	Chinese Angelica	12g
Gui Zhi	Cinnamon Twig	9g
Bai Shao Yao	White Peony	9g
Xi Xin	Asarum	3g
Tong Cao	Rice Paper Pith	6g
Da Zao	Jujube	5-8pcs
Zhi Gan Cao	Baked Licorice	6g

■ Preparation
Use as decoction or prepared form.

■ Pertaining Category
Channel Warming and Cold Dispelling

■ Functions
Warms the channels, dispels cold. Nourishes blood, invigorates blood circulation.

■ Indications
Blood deficiency with cold stagnation in the channels manifested as cold limbs, absence of thirst, soreness of the body and extremities, or abdominal spasms, pale tongue with white coat, a deep, thin, or faint pulse.

■ Cautions and Contraindications
It is contraindicated in cases of cold limbs due to interior heat accumulation or later stage of chilblain marked by cold turning to heat. Do not use overdose and for long term.

■ Modern Applications
Anemia, chronic arthritis, hernia, menstrual cramping pain, postdated menstruation, thrombophlebitis, chilblain, neuralgia, lumbago, etc.

Dao Chi San-Guide Out the Red Powder
Rehmannia and Akebia formula
导赤散

■ **Ingredients**

Sheng Di Huang	Dried Rehmannia	9g
Mu Tong	Akebia	9g
Dan Zhu Ye	Bland Bamboo Leaf	6g
Gan Cao	Licorice	6g

■ **Preparation**
Use as decoction or prepared form.

■ **Pertaining Category**
Clearing Heat from Zang-fu Organs

■ **Functions**
Clears heart fire, conducts heart fire downward. Unblocks urinary strangury, promotes diuresis to excrete heat. Nourishes Yin.

■ **Indications**
Heart fire leading to small intestine heat or turning to bladder damp heat manifested as irritable heat in the chest, restlessness, red face, thirst with a desire to drink cold water, ulceration on the tongue, dark, scanty, and painful urination, red tongue, with yellow greasy coat, a rapid pulse.

■ **Cautions and Contraindications**
Use with caution for patients with spleen and stomach deficiency. Do not use ocerdose and for long term.

■ **Modern Applications**
Acute UTI, cystitis, urethritis, acute pyelonephritis, stomatitis, etc.

Dao Tan Tang-Guide Out Phlegm Decoction
The Phlegm Resolving Decoction
导痰汤

■ **Ingredients**

Ban Xia	Pinellia Tuber	6g
Tian Nan Xing	Arisaema Tuber	3g
Zhi Shi	Immature Citrus	3g
Fu Ling	Hoelen/Poria	3g
Chen Pi	Tangerine Peel	3g
Sheng Jiang	Fresh Ginger	3g
Gan Cao	Licorice	2g

■ **Preparation**
Use as decoction or prepared form.

■ **Pertaining Category**
Dampness Drying and Phlegm Resolving

■ **Functions**
Dries dampness, resolves phlegm, stops coughing. Moves Qi, relieves stagnation.

■ **Indications**
Profuse phlegm-dampness affecting the lungs or misting the orifices manifested as cough with excessive white sputum, a fullness sensation in the chest and diaphragm, nausea, poor appetite, headache, dizziness, or coma, white greasy tongue coat, a slippery pulse.

■ **Cautions and Contraindications**
It is contraindicated during pregnancy. Use with caution for patients with weak constitution.

■ **Modern Applications**
Chronic bronchitis, trachitis, pulmonary emphysema, goiter, Meniere's syndrome, or loss of consciousness, etc.

Di Huang Yin Zi-Rehmannia Beverage
Rehmannia and Morinda Combination
地黄饮子

- **Ingredients**

Shu Di Huang	Cooked Rehmannia	6g
Ba Ji Tian	Morinda Root	6g
Shan Zhu Yu	Dogwood Fruit	6g
Shi Hu	Dendrobium	6g
Rou Cong Rong	Cistanche	6g
Fu Zi	Prepared Aconite	6g
Rou Gui	Cinnamon Bark	6g
Wu Wei Zi	Schisandra Fruit	6g
Fu Ling	Hoelen/Poria	6g
Mai Men Dong	Ophiopogon	6g
Shi Chang Pu	Sweetflag Rhizome	6g
Yuan Zhi	Polygala	6g
Sheng Jiang	Fresh Ginger	5slices
Da Zao	Jujube	1pc
Bo He	Peppermint	5-7 leaf

- **Preparation**

Use as decoction or prepared form.

- **Pertaining Category**

Internal Wind Extinguishing

- **Functions**

Nourishes the kidney Yin, tonifies the kidney Yang. Transforms phlegm, opens orifices.

■ Indications

Kidney Yin and Yang deficiency with phlegm blocking the orifices manifested as stiff tongue with slurred or loss of speech, disability or paralysis of lower limbs, dry mouth without desire to drink, red or normal colored tongue with yellow greasy coat, a deep, thin, and weak pulse.

■ Cautions and Contraindications

It is contraindicated in cases of excess patterns or liver Yang raising. Do not use for long term unless it is modified.

■ Modern Applications

Myelitis, hypertensive encephalopathy, cerebral arteriosclerosis, sequelae of cerebrovascular accident, aphasia, paralysis of the legs, syringobulbia, etc.

Di Tan Tang-Phlegm Flushing Decoction
Arisaema and Acorus Combination
涤痰汤

■ Ingredients

Ban Xia	Pinellia Tuber	8g
Fu Ling	Hoelen/Poria	6g
Dan Nan Xing	Arisaema Tuber	8g
Chen Pi	Tangerine Peel	6g
Zhi Shi	Immature Citrus	6g
Ren Shen	Ginseng	3g
Shi Chang Pu	Sweetflag Rhizome	3g
Zhu Ru	Bamboo Shavings	2g
Sheng Jiang	Fresh Ginger	3g
Da Zao	Jujube	2pcs
Gan Cao	Licorice	2g

■ Preparation

Use as decoction or prepared form.

■ **Pertaining Category**

Dampness Drying and Phlegm Resolving

■ **Functions**

Transforms and dispels phlegm, opens the orifices. Tonifies Qi.

■ **Indications**

Phlegm misting the heart orifices or with internal liver wind manifested as headache, dizziness, vertigo, stiffness of the tongue, impaired speech, rigid tongue with white or yellowish greasy coat, a slippery, wiry pulse.

■ **Cautions and Contraindications**

It is contraindicated during pregnancy. Use with caution for patients with weak constitution.

■ **Modern Applications**

Aphasia, cerebrovascular accident, seizures, bronchitis, bronchial asthma, bronchiectasis, chronic obstructive pulmonary diseases, etc.

Ding Chuan Tang-Arrest Wheezing Decoction

Ma-huang and Ginkgo Combination

定喘汤

■ **Ingredients**

Bai Guo	Ginkgo	21pcs/9g
Ma Huang	Ephedra	9g
Zi Su Zi	Perilla seed	6g
Kuan Dong Hua	Coltsfoot Flower	9g
Xing Ren	Apricot Seed	6g
Sang Bai Pi	Malberry Rootbark	9g
Huang Qin	Scute	6g
Ban Xia	Pinellia Tuber	9g
Gan Cao	Licorice	3g

■ Preparation
Use as decoction or prepared form.

■ Pertaining Category
Qi Regulating(Descending)

■ Functions
Disperses the lung Qi. Clears heat. Resolves phlegm. Descends the lung Qi, relieves asthma.

■ Indications
Phlegm-heat in the lungs or with invasion of wind-cold manifested as cough and wheezing with excessive yellow thick sputum, difficulty in breathing, or aversion to cold and fever, red tongue with yellow greasy coat, a slippery, rapid pulse.

■ Cautions and Contraindications
It is contraindicated in cases of asthma and cough due to only exterior wind-cold or Qi deficiency with prolonged history and weak pulse.

■ Modern Applications
Acute bronchitis, bronchial asthma emphysema, etc.

Ding Xian Wan-Stabilizing Epilepsy Pill
Arrest Seizures Pill
定 痫 丸

■ Ingredients

Tian Ma	Gastrodia	30g
Chuan Bei Mu	Tendrilled Fritillary	30g
Ban Xia	Pinellia Tuber	30g
Fu Ling	Hoelen/Poria	30g
Fu Shen	Hoelen/Poria	30g
Dan Nan Xing	Arisaema Tuber	15g
Shi Chang Pu	Sweetflag Rhizome	15g
Quan Xie	Scorpion	15g
Jiang Can	Bombyx	15g
Hu Po	Amber	15g
Deng Xin Cao	Rush Pith	15g
Chen Pi	Tangerine Peel	20g
Yuan Zhi	Polygala	20g
Dan Shen	Salvia Root	60g
Mai Men Dong	Ophiopogon	60g
Zhu Sha	Cinnabar	9g
Zhu Li	Dried Bamboo Sap	100ml
Sheng Jiang Zhi	Fresh Ginger Juice	50ml
Gan Cao	Licorice	120g

■ Preparation
Use as prepared pills only.

■ Pertaining Category
Treating Wind-phlegm

■ Functions
Resolves and dispels phlegm, opens the sensory orifices, extinguishes wind.

■ Indications

Liver wind with phlegm-heat leading to recurrent seizures manifested as vertigo, weakness, and a stifling sensation in the chest, followed by sudden falling down with loss of consciousness, upward-rolling of eyes, spitting of mucus with a loud, raspy sound, convulsions, or incontinence of the bowels or urine, white greasy tongue coat, a wiry, slippery pulse.

■ Cautions and Contraindications

It is contraindicated during pregnancy. Do not use overdose and for long term due to toxicity of some ingredients.

■ Modern Applications

Primary or secondary epilepsy.

Ding Xiang Shi Di Tang-Cloves and Kaki Decoction
Cloves and Kaki Combination
丁 香 柿 蒂 汤

■ Ingredients

Ding Xiang	Cloves Flower-bud	6g
Shi Di	Kaki Calyx	6-9g
Ren Shen	Ginseng	3-6g
Sheng Jiang	Fresh Ginger	6-9g

■ Preparation

Use as decoction or prepared form.

■ Pertaining Category

Qi Regulating (Descending)

■ Functions

Warms the middle burner, tonifies Qi. Descends the rebellious Qi, stops hiccups.

■ Indications
Stomach Qi and Yang deficiency with rebellious stomach Qi
manifested as hiccups, belching, nausea and vomiting, fullness of
chest and epigastrium, loss of appetite, cold limbs, pale tongue with
white coat, a slow, weak pulse.

■ Cautions and Contraindications
It is contraindicated in cases of hiccups or vomiting due to excess
or deficient heat.

■ Modern Applications
Hiccups after operation due to spasm of diaphragm, morning
sickness, neurological hiccups, etc.

Ding Zhi Wan-Stabilize the Emotions Pill
定 志 丸

■ Ingredients

Ren Shen	Ginseng	90g
Fu Ling	Hoelen/Poria	90g
Shi Chang Pu	Sweetflag Rhizome	60g
Yuan Zhi	Polygala	60g

■ Preparation
Use as prepared form or decoction with properly reduced dosage.

■ Pertaining Category
Spirit Calming with Nourishing Sedative Herbs

■ Functions
Tonifies the heart Qi, sedates the heart, calms spirit.

■ Indications
Heart Qi deficiency with disturbance of spirit manifested as
palpitation, easily frightened, anxiety, insomnia, forgetfulness, pale
tongue, a weak pulse.

118

■ **Cautions and Contraindications**

Do not use for long term and during pregnancy.

■ **Modern Applications**

Anxiety, neurosis, and other psychological disorders, etc.

This formula is from "Qian Jin Yao Fang" (Thousand Ducat Formula).

Du Huo Ji Sheng Tang-Pubescent Angelica and Loranthus Decoction
Tuhuo and Vaeicum Combination
独活寄生汤

■ **Ingredients**

Du Huo	*Tuhuo*	9g
Sang Ji Sheng	*Loranthus*	6g
Du Zhong	*Eucommia Bark*	6g
Niu Xi	*Achyranthes Root*	6g
Xi Xin	*Asarum*	3g
Qin Jiao	*Big Leaf Gentiana*	6g
Fu Ling	*Hoelen/Poria*	6g
Rou Gui	*Cinnamon Bark*	6g
Fang Feng	*Siler*	6g
Chuan Xiong	*Ligusticum*	6g
Ren Shen	*Ginseng*	6g
Dang Gui	*Chinese Angelica*	6g
Bai Shao Yao	*White Peony*	6g
Sheng Di Huang	*Dried Rehmannia*	6g
Gan Cao	*Licorice*	6g

■ **Preparation**

Use as decoction or prepared form.

■ **Pertaining Category**
Wind-dampness Expelling

■ **Functions**
Expels wind-dampness, relieves pain from arthragia. Nourishes the liver and kidney, strengthens tendons and bones, tonifies Qi and blood.

■ **Indications**
Chronic bi syndrome due to wind-cold-dampness invasion with deficiency of the liver, kidney, Qi, and blood manifested as pain and coldness of lower back and knees, preference to warmth and aversion to damp-cold, difficult movement, soreness, numbness, and weakness of limbs, or joint stiffness and deformities, pale tongue with white coat, a deep, weak pulse.

■ **Cautions and Contraindications**
Xi Xin (Asarum) can not be used overdose or for a long term.

■ **Modern Applications**
Chronic osteoarthritis, lumbago, sciatica, chronic rheumatic or rheumatoid arthritis, sequelae of poliomyelitis, etc.

Du Qi Wan-Capital Qi Pill
Rehmannia and Schizandra Formula
(七味) 都气丸

■ **Ingredients**

Shu Di Huang	Cooked Rehmannia	24g
Shan Zhu Yu	Dogwood Fruit	12g
Shan Yao	Dioscorea	12g
Fu Ling	Hoelen/Poria	9g
Ze Xie	Alisma	9g
Mu Dan Pi	Moutan Bark	9g
Wu Wei Zi	Schizandra	6g

■ **Preparation**
Use as decoction or prepared form.

■ **Pertaining Category**
Yin Tonifying

■ **Functions**
Nourishes the liver and kidney Yin, assists kidney in grasping Qi.

■ **Indications**
Yin deficiency of the liver and kidney with deficient lung and kidney Qi manifested as wheezing, shortness of breath, worse on exertion, weak voice, or chronic cough, hiccup, soreness and weakness of lower back, tinnitus, red tongue with thin coat, a thin, rapid pulse.

■ **Cautions and Contraindications**
Use with extreme caution for patients with indigestion and diarrhea due to deficiency of the spleen and stomach.

■ **Modern Applications**
Asthma, bronchial asthma, chronic bronchitis, pulmonary emphysema, pulmonary tuberculosis, etc.

E Jiao Ji Zi Huang Tang-Donkey-hide Gelatin and Egg Yolk Decoction
Ass-hide Gelatin and Egg Yolk Decoction
阿 胶 鸡 子 黄 汤

Ingredients

E Jiao	Equus/Gelatin	6g
Bai Shao Yao	White Peony	9g
Shi Jue Ming	Abalone	15g
Gou Teng	Uncaria	6g
Sheng Di Huang	Dried Rehmannia	12g
Mu Li	Oyster Shell	12g
Luo Shi Teng	Trachelospermum	9g
Fu Shen	Hoelen/Poria	12g
Ji Zi Huang	Egg Yolk	2pcs
Zhi Gan Cao	Baked Licorice	1.8g

■ Preparation

Use as decoction. E Jiao should be dissolved separately in boiling water and added into the strained decoction. Egg Yolks are boiled hard and mixed with the strained decoction. Shi Jue Ming should be decocted first.

■ Pertaining Category

Internal Wind Extinguishing

■ Functions

Nourishes Yin and blood, suppresses the liver Yang, extinguishes wind.

■ Indications

Endogenous wind due to Yin and blood deficiency with liver Yang raising manifested as twitches and spasms of muscles, or rigid extremities, trembling of hands, dizziness, blurred vision, dark red tongue with scanty coat, a thin, rapid pulse.

■ Cautions and Contraindications

None noted.

■ Modern Applications

Encephalitis, meningitis, hepatic coma, Parkinson's disease, etc.

Er Chen Tang-Two Matured Ingredients Decoction
Citrus and Pinellia Combination
二 陈 汤

■ **Ingredients**

Ban Xia	Pinellia Tuber	15g
Chen Pi	Tangerine Peel	15g
Fu Ling	Hoelen/Poria	9g
Zhi Gan Cao	Baked Licorice	5g
Sheng Jiang	Fresh Ginger	3g
Wu Mei	Black Plum	1pc

■ **Preparation**

Use as decoction or prepared form.

■ **Pertaining Category**

Dampness Drying and Phlegm Resolving

■ **Functions**

Dries dampness, resolves phlegm. Moves Qi, harmonizes middle burner.

■ **Indications**

Phlegm-dampness obstructing Qi in the upper and middle burners manifested as cough with excessive white sputum, a fullness sensation in the chest and epigastrium, nausea, vomiting, palpitation, dizziness, lassitude, white and moist tongue coat, a slippery pulse.

■ **Cautions and Contraindications**

It is contraindicated in cases of dry cough or coughing of blood due to Yin deficiency.

■ **Modern Applications**

Chronic bronchitis, gastritis, peptic ulcer, goiter, Miniere's syndrome, etc.

Er Dong Tang-Two Winter Decoction
Ophiopogon and Asparagus Decoction
二冬汤

■ **Ingredients**

Mai Men Dong	Ophiopogon	12g
Tian Men Dong	Asparagus	12g
Tian Hua Fen	Trichosanthes	12g
Huang Qin	Scute	9g
Zhi Mu	Anemarrhena	12g
Gan Cao	Licorice	6g
Ren Shen	Ginseng	6g
He Ye	Lotus Leaf	3g

■ **Preparation**
Use as decoction or prepared form.

■ **Pertaining Category**
Yin Tonifying

■ **Functions**
Nourishes the lung and kidney Yin, tonifies Qi. Clears heat from upper burner, relieves thirst.

■ **Indications**
Diabetes due to Yin and Qi deficiency of the lung and kidney with heat in the upper burner manifested as excessive thirst, frequent urination, lassitude, dry mouth, red tip tongue with scanty coat, a thin, weak, and rapid pulse.

■ **Cautions and Contraindications**
None noted.

■ **Modern Applications**
Diabetes, pulmonary tuberculosis, etc.

Er Long Zuo Ci Wan-Pill for Deafness That Is Kind to the Left

Deafness Left(Kidney Yin)-Benefiting Pill

耳聋左慈丸

■ **Ingredients**

Shu Di Huang	Cooked Rehmannia	24g
Shan Yao	Dioscorea	12g
Shan Zhu Yu	Dogwood Fruit	12g
Mu Dan Pi	Moutan Bark	9g
Fu Ling	Hoelen/Poria	9g
Ze Xie	Alisma	9g
Ci Shi	Magnetite	24g
Wu Wei Zi	Schisandra	6g
Shi Chang Pu	Sweetflag Rhizome	6g

■ **Preparation**

Use as decoction or prepared form.

■ **Pertaining Category**

Yin Tonifying

■ **Functions**

Nouishes the kidney Yin and essence, descends deficient fire, benefits ears.

■ **Indications**

Kidney Yin and essence deficiency with hearing problems manifested as tinnitus, or deafness, or hearing loss in the elderly, soreness and weakness of lower back and knees, dry mouth, malar flash, red tongue with scanty coat, a thin, weak, and rapid pulse.

Cautions and Contraindications

Use with caution in cases of indigestion or diarrhea with white and greasy tongue coat due to spleen deficiency and dampness retention.

Modern Applications

Tinnitus, deafness, Meniere's syndrome, diabetes, etc.

Er Miao San-Two Mysterious Powder
Two Marvel Powder
二 妙 散

Ingredients

Huang Bai	*Phellodendron*	15g
Cang Zhu	*Atractylodes*	15g

Preparation

Use as prepared form or decoction with properly reduced dosage.

Pertaining Category

Damp-heat Clearing

Functions

Clears heat, dries dampness.

Indications

Damp-heat in the lower burner manifested as lower back pain, painful, red, hot, swollen knees and feet, or weakness of lower limbs, yellow and odorous vaginal discharge, eczema, dark, yellow and scanty urine, red tongue with yellow greasy coat, a slippery, rapid pulse.

- **Cautions and Contraindications**
None noted.

- **Modern Applications**
Acute or chronic UTI, vaginitis, cervicitis, rheumatic, rheumatoid, or gouty arthritis, beriberi, etc.

Er Xian Tang-Two Immortals Decoction
Curculigo and Epimedium Combination
二仙汤

- **Ingredients**

Xian Mao	*Curculigo*	9-15g
Xian Ling Pi	*Epimedium*	9-15g
Dang Gui	*Chinese Angelica*	9-12g
Ba Ji Tian	*Morinda Root*	6-9g
Huang Bai	*Phellodendron Bark*	6-9g
Zhi Mu	*Anemarrhena*	6-9g

- **Preparation**
Use as decoction or prepared form.

- **Pertaining Category**
Additional Formulas for Ob-Gyn Disorders

- **Functions**
Warms the kidney Yang, nourishes the kidney essence and Yin. Drains deficient fire from lower burner. Regulates Chong and Ren channels.

■ **Indications**

Pre and post menopausal syndrome or chronic diseases with kidney Yin, Yang, and essence deficiency manifested as menstrual disturbances, hot flushes, sweating, nervousness, dizziness, fatigue, irritability, insomnia, palpitation, depression, frequent urination, soreness and weakness of lower back and knees, light red tongue with scanty coat, a thin, weak, or rapid pulse.

■ **Cautions and Contraindications**

None noted.

■ **Modern Applications**

Menopausal syndrome, hyperthyroidism, primary hypertension, chronic glomerulonephritis, chronic pyelonephritis, chronic UTI, etc.

Er Zhi Wan-Two Ultimate Pill
Eclipta and Ligustrum Combination
二至丸

■ **Ingredients**

| Han Lian Cao | *Eclipta* | 10-15g |
| Nu Zhen Zi | *Ligustrum* | 10-15g |

■ **Preparation**

Use as prepared form or decoction.

■ **Pertaining Category**

Yin Tonifying

■ **Functions**

Nourishes the kidney and liver Yin.

Indications

Yin deficiency of the liver and kidney manifested as dizziness, blurred vision, tinnitus, dry throat, a bitter taste in the mouth, soreness and weakness of lower back and knees, insomnia or dream disturbed sleep, nocturnal emission, or early graying of hair, red and dry tongue with scanty coat, a thin, rapid pulse.

Cautions and Contraindications

None noted.

Modern Applications

Baldness, menopausal condition, vertigo, neurasthenia, etc.

Fang Feng Tang-Ledebouriella Decoction
Siler Combination
防 风 汤

Ingredients

Fang Feng	Siler	9g
Dang Gui	Chinese Angelica	9g
Chi Fu Ling	(Red)Hoelen/Poria	9g
Xing Ren	Apricot Seed	6g
Huang Qin	Scute	3g
Qin Jiao	Big Leaf Gentiana	9g
Ma Huang	Ephedra	9g
Rou Gui	Cinnamon Bark	6g
Sheng Jiang	Fresh Ginger	6g
Gan Cao	Licorice	6g
Da Zao	Jujube	3pcs

Preparation

Use as decoction or prepared form.

Pertaining Category

Wind-dampness Expelling

■ **Functions**

Expels wind-cold-dampness, unblocks channels and collaterals, alleviates pain.

■ **Indications**

Win-cold-damp bi syndrome with predominant wind manifested as migrating joint pain, difficult joint flexion and extension in the limbs, or aversion to wind-cold and fever, thin white tongue coat, a superficial, slippery pulse.

■ **Cautions and Contraindications**

Use cautiously for patients with constitutional Yin deficiency, or with hypertension and heart problems. Do not use for long term.

■ **Modern Applications**

Rheumatic fever, rheumatic arthritis, etc.

Fang Feng Tong Sheng San-Siler Magical Unblocking Powder
Siler and Platycodon Formula
防 风 通 圣 散

■ Ingredients

Fang Feng	*Siler*	15g
Jing Jie	*Schizonepeta*	15g
Lian Qiao	*Forsythia*	15g
Ma Huang	*Ephedra*	15g
Bo He	*Peppermint*	15g
Chuan Xiong	*Ligusticum*	15g
Dang Gui	*Chinese Angelica*	15g
Bai Shao Yao	*White Peony*	15g
Bai Zhu	*White Atractylodes*	15g
Zhi Zi	*Gardenia Fruit*	15g
Da Huang	*Rhubarb*	15g
Mang Xiao	*Mirabilitum*	15g
Shi Gao	*Gypsum*	30g
Huang Qin	*Scute*	30g
Jie Geng	*Platycodon*	30g
Hua Shi	*Talcum*	90g
Gan Cao	*Licorice*	60g
Sheng Jiang	*Fresh Ginger*	3slices

■ Preparation
Use as prepared form (powder, pill, etc.), or decoction with properly reducesd dosage.

■ Pertaining Category
Relieving Both Exterior and Interior

■ Functions
Expels wind, releases the exterior. Eliminates interior intense heat, promotes bowel movement.

■ Indications

Exterior wind-heat with intense heat in the Qi level and Yangming Fu organs manifested as chills and fever, headache, dizziness, red, swelling, and painful eyes, a bitter taste in the mouth, dry mouth, sore throat, a stifling sensation in the chest, cough, difficulty in breathing, thick-sticky mucus, constipation, dark and scanty urine, skin ulcers and rashes, hemorrhoids, red tongue with yellow coat, a rapid, forceful pulse.

■ Cautions and Contraindications

It is contraindicated for patients with weak constitution.

■ Modern Applications

Upper respiratory infection, influenza, acute conjunctivitis, erysipelas, food poisoning, carbuncle, sore, urticaria, dermatitis, acne, obesity, etc.

Fang Ji Huang Qi Tang-Stephania and Astragalus Decoction
Stephania and Astragalus Combination
防己黄芪汤

■ Ingredients

Fang Ji	Stephania Root	12g
Huang Qi	Astragalus	15g
Bai Zhu	White Atractylodes	9g
Gan Cao	Licorice	6g
Sheng Jiang	Fresh Ginger	4slices
Da Zao	Jujube	1pc

■ Preparation

Use as decoction or prepared form.

■ Pertaining Category

Downward Dampness Draining

132

■ Functions

Tonifies Qi, strengthens the spleen. Expels wind, promotes urination, reduces edema.

■ Indications

Wind-damp edema with spleen and defensive Qi deficiency manifested as superficial edema, difficult urination, or retention of urine, heaviness of body, sweating, aversion to wind, pale tongue with white coat, a superficial pulse.

■ Cautions and Contraindications

It is contraindicated for excess type of edema. Do not use overdose and for long term.

■ Modern Applications

Acute glomerulonephritis, chronic nephrotic syndrome, rheumatic heart disease, etc.

Fei Er Wan-Fat Baby Pill
Nourish the Baby Formula
肥 儿 丸

■ Ingredients

Shen Qu	Medicated Leaven	300g
Huang Lian	Coptis	300g
Rou Dou Kou	Nutmeg	150g
Shi Jun Zi	Quisqualis Fruit	150g
Mai Ya	Barley Sprout	150g
Bing Lang	Betel Nut	120g
Mu Xiang	Saussurea	60g

■ Preparation

Use as prepared form.

■ Pertaining Category

Parasites Expelling

Functions

Kills parasites, relieves food stagnation. Strengthens the spleen. Clears the stomach heat.

Indications

Malnutrition due to parasites accumulation with spleen deficiency and stomach heat manifested as sallow complexion, emaciation, abdominal distention and pain, nausea or vomiting after eating, bad breath, indigestion, loose stools or diarrhea, low grade fever, pale red tongue, a weak, rapid pulse.

Cautions and Contraindications

Do not use for long term.

Modern Applications

Ascariasis, malnutrition and indigestion in children, etc.

Fu Ling Pi Tang-Hoelen Peel Decoction
Poria Combination
茯苓皮汤

Ingredients

Fu Ling Pi	Hoelen/Poria Peel	15g
Yi Yi Ren	Coix Seed	15g
Zhu Ling	Polyporu	9g
Da Fu Pi	Areca Peel	9g
Tong Cao	Rice Paper Pith	9g
Dan Zhu Ye	Bland Bamboo Leaf	6g

Preparation

Use as decoction or prepared form.

Pertaining Category

Damp-heat Clearing

■ Functions
Promotes urination, drains damp-heat.

■ Indications
Damp-heat in the middle and lower burners manifested as difficult or retention of urine, thirst with a desire to drink only a little fluids, a fullness sensation in the lower abdomen, or constipation, heavy and distended head, heavy and aching of the body, yellow or white greasy tongue coat, a soft, rapid pulse.

■ Cautions and Contraindications
Do not use for long term..

■ Modern Applications
Acute UTI, cystitis, prostatitis, etc.

Fu Yuan Huo Xue Tang-Invigorate Blood Decoction for Recovery
Tang-kuei and Persica Combination
复 元 活 血 汤

■ Ingredients

Chai Hu	Bupleurum	15g
Tian Hua Fen	Trichosanthes Root	9g
Dang Gui Wei	Chinese Angelica	9g
Hong Hua	Safflower	6g
Chuan Shan Jia	Pangolin Scales	6g
Jiu Da Huang	Rhubarb	30g
Tao Ren	Peach Kernel	9g
Gan Cao	Licorice	6g

■ Preparation
Use as decoction or prepared form. Rhubarb is prepared with wine.

■ **Pertaining Category**
Blood Invigorating

■ **Functions**
Promotes blood circulation, removes blood stasis. Soothes the liver, unblocks the channels.

■ **Indications**
Blood stasis and Qi stagnation in the hypochondrium due to trauma manifested as unbearable stabbing pain in the chest and flanks, bruises, swelling, purple tongue, a wiry, hesitant pulse.

■ **Cautions and Contraindications**
It is contraindicated during pregnancy and in cases of excessive menstrual bleeding, bleeding diathesis, or any bleeding disorders. Use with extreme caution for patients with weak constitution.

■ **Modern Applications**
Pain and swelling due to traumatic injury, contusion in the chest and costal region, intercostal neuralgia, costal chondritis, acute lumbar sprain, etc.

Fu Zi Li Zhong Wan (Tang)-Regulate the Middle Burner Pill (Tang) with Aconite
Aconite, Ginseng, and Ginger Combination
附 子 理 中 丸 (汤)

■ **Ingredients**

Pao Fu Zi	Prepared Aconite	6g
Ren Shen	Ginseng	9g
Bai Zhu	White Atractylodes	9g
Gan Jiang	Dried Ginger	9g
Zhi Gan Cao	Baked Licorice	6g

136

■ Preparation
Use as decoction or prepared form.

■ Pertaining Category
Middle Burner Warming and Cold Dispelling

■ Functions
Strongly warmsYang, dispels cold. Tonifies the spleen and stomach Qi.

■ Indications
Severe Yang deficiency of the spleen and stomach with internal cold manifested as fullness and pain in the epigastric and abdominal regions which are alleviated by warmth and pressure, absence of thirst, watery diarrhea, vomiting of clear fluid, cold limbs, or spasms of caff muscles, pale tongue with white coat, a deep, fainting, and slow pulse.

■ Cautions and Contraindications
It is contraindicated in cases of exterior wind-heat invasion or interior heat with Yin deficiency.

■ Modern Applications
Chronic gastroenteritis, peptic ulcer, chronic colitis, gastroptosis, indigestion, cholera, etc.

Gan Cao Xie Xin Tang-Licorice Decoction to Purge the Stomach
Pinellia and Licorice Combination
甘草泻心汤

■ Ingredients

Ban Xia	Pinellia Tuber	9g
Huang Qin	Scute	6g
Gan Jiang	Dried Ginger	6g
Ren Shen	Ginseng	6g
Huang Lian	Coptis	3g
Zhi Gan Cao	Baked Licorice	9-12g
Da Zao	Jujube	4pcs

■ Preparation
Use as decoction or prepared form.

■ Pertaining Category
Regulating the Intestines and Stomach (Mediating)

■ Functions
Tonifies Qi. Harmonizes the stomach, descends the rebellious stomach Qi downward, stops vomiting. Relieves focal distention.

■ Indications
Disharmony between stomach and intestines with stomach Qi deficiency manifested as fullness and hardness in the epigastrium, retching, irritability, loud borborygmus, diarrhea with undigested food in the stool, abdominal distention, thin yellow tongue coat, a weak, slightly wiry or slippery pulse.

■ Cautions and Contraindications
It is contraindicated in cases of retching and nausea due to stomach Yin deficiency.

■ Modern Applications
Acute or chronic gastroenteritis, peptic ulcer, indigestion, gastrointestinal neurosis, morning sickness, etc.
This formula is modified from Ban Xia Xie Xin Tang (Pinellia Decoction to Purge the Stomach).

Gan Jiang Ling Zhu Tang-Licorice, Dried Ginger, Hoelen, and Atractylodes Decoction

Licorice, Ginger, Poria, and Atractylodes Combination

甘姜苓术汤

■ Ingredients

Gan Jiang	*Dried Ginger*	12g
Fu Ling	*Hoelen/Poria*	12g
Bai Zhu	*White Atractylodes*	9g
Gan Cao	*Licorice*	6g

■ Preparation
Use as decoction or prepared form.

■ Pertaining Category
Additional Formulas for Internal Medicine

■ Functions
Dispels cold, transforms dampness. Warms channels, clears collaterals.

■ Indications
Obstruction of channels and collaterals in the lower back due to damp-cold invasion manifested as cold pain and heaviness of the lower back with difficulty turning waist, pain reduced by applying heat, but not relieved by lying down and resting, pain aggravated during cold and rainy weather, white greasy tongue coat, a deep, soft, and slow pulse.

■ Cautions and Contraindications
None noted.

■ Modern Applications
Lower back pain, rheumatic or rheumatoid arthritis, etc.

Gan Lu Xiao Du Dan-Sweet Dew Toxin Eliminating Elixir

Talc and Scute Formula

甘露消毒丹

■ **Ingredients**

Hua Shi	Talcum	450g
Yin Chen Hao	Oriental Wormwood	330g
Huang Qin	Scute	300g
Shi Chang Pu	Sweetflag Rhizome	180g
Chuan Bei Mu	Tendrilled Fritillary	150g
Mu Tong	Akebia	150g
Huo Xiang	Agastache	120g
She Gan	Belamcanda	120g
Lian Qiao	Forsythia Fruit	120g
Bo He	Peppermint	120g
Bai Dou Kou	Cluster Fruit	120g

■ **Preparation**
Use as prepared form or decoction with properly reduced dosage.

■ **Pertaining Category**
Damp-heat Clearing

■ **Functions**
Drains dampness, resolves turbidity. Clears heat, relieves toxicity.

■ **Indications**
Toxic damp-heat or seasonal epidemic damp-heat retaining in the Qi level manifested as fever, lassitude, lethargy, aching and heaviness of limbs, facial and throat swollen, a stifling sensation in the chest, abdominal distention, bright yellowish skin, thirst, vomiting, diarrhea, dark, scanty, and difficult urination, red tongue with white or yellow greasy coat, a slippery, rapid pulse.

■ **Cautions and Contraindications**

It is contraindicated in cases of vomiting and diarrhea due to deficiency of the spleen and stomach. Do not use overdose or for long term.

■ **Modern Applications**

Acute gastroenteritis, acute infectious hepatitis, cholecystitis, pyelonephritis, acute UTI, mild case of encephalitis B, etc.

Gan Mai Da Zao Tang-Licorice, Wheat Chaff, and Jujube Decoction
Licorice and Jujube Combination
甘 麦 大 枣 汤

■ **Ingredients**

Gan Cao	Licorice	9g
Fu Xiao Mai	Wheat Chaff	9-15g
Da Zao	Jujube	5-7pcs

■ **Preparation**

Use as decoction or prepared form.

■ **Pertaining Category**

Spirit Calming with Nourishing Sedative Herbs

■ **Functions**

Nourishes the heart, calms spirit. Harmonizes the middle burner, tonifies the spleen Qi. Relieves spasms.

■ **Indications**

Deficiency of the heart and spleen with stagnant liver Qi manifested as hysteria, disorientation, moody, crying easily, restlessness, insomnia, frequent yawning, or abnormal speech and behavior, slight red tongue with thin white or scanty coat, a wiry, thin, and rapid pulse. mild anxiety

■ **Cautions and Contraindications**
None noted.

■ **Modern Applications**
Hysteria, mania, neurosis, neurasthenia, etc.

Ge Gen Huang Qin Huang Lian Tang-
Pueraria, Scute, and Coptis Decoction
Pueraria, Scute, and Coptis Combination
葛 根 黄 芩 黄 连 汤

■ **Ingredients**

Ge Gen	*Pueraria*	15g
Huang Qin	*Scute*	9g
Huang Lian	*Coptis*	6-9g
Zhi Gan Cao	*Baked Licorice*	6g

■ **Preparation**
Use as decoction or prepared form.

■ **Pertaining Category**
Relieving Both Exterior and Interior

■ **Functions**
Expels wind-heat, releases the exterior. Eliminates internal heat in the stomach and intestines.

■ **Indications**
Exterior wind-heat with large intestine damp-heat manifested as fever, or slight chills, diarrhea with foul odor, a burning sensation in the anus, irritable heat in the chest and epigastrium, thirst with dry mouth, red tongue with yellow coat, a rapid pulse.

Cautions and Contraindications

It is contraindicated in cases of diarrhea due to cold or deficiency.

Modern Applications

Acute gastroenteritis, early stage of dysentery, early stage of amoebic dysentery, acute colitis, common cold, etc.

Ge Gen Tang-Pueraria Decoction
Pueraria Combination
葛根汤

Ingredients

Ge Gen	Pueraria Root	12g
Ma Huang	Ephedra	6g
Gui Zhi	Cinnamon Twig	6g
Bai Shao Yao	White Peony	6g
Sheng Jiang	Fresh Ginger	9g
Da Zao	Jujube	4pcs
Zhi Gan Cao	Baked Licorice	6g

Preparation

Use as decoction or prepared form.

Pertaining Category

Pungent Warm Exterior Relieving

Functions

Expels wind-cold, releases the exterior and muscle layer, relieves muscle-ache of the neck. Promotes generation of fluids.

Indications

Wind-cold invasion obstructing Taiyang channel manifested as aversion to wind-cold, fever, absence of sweating, stiffness and pain of neck and upper back, thin white tongue coat, a superficial, tight pulse.

■ Cautions and Contraindications

It is contraindicated in cases of exterior deficiency with spontaneous sweating, exterior wind-heat, and weak constitution. Use with caution for patients with hypertension and heart problems.

■ Modern Applications

Common cold, headache, neck stiffness and pain, frozen shoulder, etc.

This formula is modified from Ma Huang Tang (Ephedra Decoction).

Ge Xia Zhu Yu Tang-Romove Blood Stasis below the Diaphragm Decoction
Persica and Carthamus Combination
膈下逐瘀汤

■ Ingredients

Dang Gui	Chinese Angelica	9g
Chuan Xiong	Ligusticum	6g
Tao Ren	Peach Kernel	9g
Hong Hua	Safflower	9g
Mu Dan Pi	Moutan Bark	6g
Chi Shao Yao	Red Peony	6g
Wu Ling Zhi	Trogopterus	9g
Yan Hu Suo	Corydalis	3g
Wu Yao	Lindera	6g
Xiang Fu	Cyperus Tuber	5g
Zhi Ke	Bitter Orange	5g
Gan Cao	Licorice	9g

■ Preparation

Use as decoction or prepared form. Wu Ling Zhi should be wrapped in gauze when making decoction.

■ **Pertaining Category**
Blood Invigorating

■ **Functions**
Promotes the circulation of blood and Qi, removes blood stasis, relieves pain.

■ **Indications**
Blood stasis below the diaphragm manifested as palpable mass under the diaphragm, hypochondriac piercing pain, infantile abdominal mass with fixed pain, or a feeling of abdominal heaviness, purple tongue, a wiry, hesitant pulse.

■ **Cautions and Contraindications**
It is contraindicated during pregnancy and in cases of excessive menstrual bleeding, bleeding diathesis, or any bleeding disorders, etc.

■ **Modern Applications**
Dysmenorrhea, amenorrhea, irregular menstruation, abdominal mass, cirrhosis of liver, etc.

Gu Ben Zhi Beng Tang-Secure Root and Stop Uterine Bleeding Decoction
固 本 止 崩 汤

■ **Ingredients**

Shu Di Huang	Cooked Rehmannia	18g
Bai Zhu	White Atractylodes	9g
Huang Qi	Astragalus	15g
Dang Gui	Chinese Angelica	6g
Ren Shen	Ginseng	9g
Pao Jiang	Blast-fried Ginger	6g

■ **Preparation**
Use as decoction or prepared form.

■ **Pertaining Category**
Additional Formulas for Ob-Gyn Disorders

■ **Functions**
Tonifies the spleen Qi, secures blood, stops bleeding.

■ **Indications**
Spleen Qi deficiency leading to uncontrolled uterine bleeding with pale colored blood and thin quality, shortness of breath, listlessness, pale complexion, cold limbs, poor appetite, or edema of face and limbs, pale swollen tongue with thin white coat, a deep, weak pulse.

■ **Cautions and Contraindications**
None noted.

■ **Modern Applications**
Uterine bleeding, menorrhagia, polymenorrhea, etc.
For best results, omit Dang Gui, add Shan Yao(Chinese Wild Yam Root)12g, Sheng Ma (Cimicifuga) 3g, Wu Zei Gu (Cuttle-fish Bone)9g, Da Zao (Jujube) 8pcs.

Gu Chong Tang-Stabilize Gushing Decoction
固冲汤

■ **Ingredients**

Huang Qi	Astragalus	18g
Bai Zhu	White Atractylodes	30g
Long Gu	Dragon Bone	24g
Mu Li	Oyster Shell	24g
Shan Zhu Yu	Dogwood Fruit	24g
Bai Shao Yao	White Peony	12g
Hai piao Xiao	Cuttle-fish Bone	12g
Qian Cao Gen	Madder Root	9g
Zong Lu Tan	Trachycarpus	6g
Wu Bei Zi	Rhus/Melaphis	1.5g

■ Preparation
Use as decoction or prepared form.

■ Pertaining Category
Stablizing the Menses and Stopping Leukorrhea

■ Functions
Tonifies the spleen Qi, stabilizes the penetrating vessel, stops bleeding.

■ Indications
Spleen Qi deficiency with inability to control blood manifested as uterine bleeding or excessive menstruation with pale colored blood and thin quality, palpitation, shortness of breath, poor appetite, loose stools, pale tongue, a thin, weak pulse.

■ Cautions and Contraindications
It is improper to use this formula for bleeding due to excess heat. It needs to be modified for unstable condition such as profuse sweating, cold limbs, faint and imperceptible pulse due to loss of blood.

■ Modern Applications
Menorrhagia, functional uterine bleeding, excessive postpartum bleeding, bleeding peptic ulcer, etc.

Gu Jing Wan-Stabilize the Menses Pill
固 经 丸

■ Ingredients

Huang Qin	Scute	30g
Bai Shao Yao	White Peony	30g
Gui Ban	Tortoise Plastron	30g
Chun Pi	Ailanthus Bark	21g
Huang Bai	Phellodendron	9g
Xiang Fu	Cyperus Tuber	7.5g

- **Preparation**

Use as prepared form or decoction with properly reduced dosage.

- **Pertaining Category**

Stabilizing the Menses and Stopping Leukorrhea

- **Functions**

Nourishes Yin, clears heat. Stabilizes menses, stops bleeding.

- **Indications**

Yin deficiency with internal heat manifested as prolonged menstrual period that alternates between trickling and gushing of blood, marked by dark red or purple, thick sticky or with clots, irritable heat in the chest, malar flush, abdominal pain, dark scanty urine, constipation, red tongue with scanty coat, a wiry, rapid, and thin pulse.

- **Cautions and Contraindications**

None noted.

- **Modern Applications**

Menorrhagia, functional uterine bleeding, irregular menstruation, etc.

Gua Di San-Melon Pedicle Powder
Melon Pedicle Formula
瓜蒂散

- **Ingredients**

| Gua Di | *Cucumis* | 1-3g |
| Chi Xiao Dou | *Phaseolus* | 1-3g |

- **Preparation**

Grind both ingredients into powder, taken with decoction of Dan Dou Chi (Prepared Soybean 6-9g).

- **Pertaining Category**

Inducing Vomiting

- **Functions**

Induces vomiting to eliminate phlegm and stagnant food.

- **Indications**

Phlegm and food retention obstructing in the chest and epigastrium manifested as a fullness and stuffiness sensation with firm areas in the chest and epigastrium, irritability, difficult breathing due to a feeling of Qi ascending into the throat, greasy tongue coat, a slight superficial pulse in the first (Cun) position.

- **Cautions and Contraindications**

Do not use during pregnancy. Use with extreme caution for patients with weak constitution.

- **Modern Applications**

Early stage of food poisoning, poisoning due to drug, hepatitis, etc. *This formula is from "Shang Han Lun" (Treatise on Febrile Diseases).*

Gua Lou Xie Bai Bai Jiu Tang-Trichosanthes, Macrostem Onion, and White Wine Decoction
瓜蒌薤白白酒汤

- **Ingredients**

Gua Lou	Trichosanthes Fruit	12g
Xie Bai	Macrostem Onion	9-12g
Bai Jiu	White Wine	30-60ml

- **Preparation**

Use as decoction or prepared form.

■   **Pertaining Category**
Qi Regulating(Moving)

■   **Functions**
Circulates Yang Qi in the chest, expands the chest. Resolves phlegm disperses obstruction.

■   **Indications**
Phlegm obstructing Qi and blood circulation in the chest manifested as pain with a stifling sensation in the chest, even radiating to the back, cough with sputum, difficulty in breathing, shortness of breath, white greasy tongue coat, a deep, wiry, or tight pulse.

■   **Cautions and Contraindications**
It is contraindicated in cases of chest pain due to phlegm-heat or with lung Yin deficiency. Reduce the amount of liquor if the patient is not good at drinking wine.

■   **Modern Applications**
Angina pectoris of coronary heart disease, non-suppurative costal chondritis, intercostal neuralgia, chronic bronchitis, etc.

Gua Lou Xie Bai Ban Xia Tang-
Trichosanthes, Macrostem Onion, and
Pinellia Decoction
Trichosanthes, Bakeri, and Pinellia Combination
瓜蒌薤白半夏汤

■   **Ingredients**

Gua Lou	Trichosanthes Fruit	12g
Xie Bai	Macrostem Onion	9-12g
Bai Jiu	White Wine	30-60ml
Ban Xia	Pinellia Tuber	9-12g

■ Preparation
Use as decoction or prepared form.

■ Pertaining Category
Qi Regulating(Moving)

■ Functions
Circulates Yang Qi in the chest, expands the chest. Resolves phlegm, unblocks the obstruction.

■ Indications
Severe phlegm accumulating in the chest blocking Qi, blood, and Yang circulation manifested as severe chest pain radiating to the back, shoulder, and down to the arm, shortness of breath, difficulty in lying down comfortably, pale or purplish tongue with white greasy moist coat, a wiry, slippery pulse.

■ Cautions and Contraindications
It is contraindicated in cases of chest pain due to phlegm-heat or with lung Yin deficiency. Reduce the amount of liquor if the patient is not good at drinking wine.

■ Modern Applications
Angina pectoris of coronary heart disease, non-suppurative costal chondritis, intercostal neuralgia, chronic bronchitis, etc.

Gui Lu Er Xian Jiao-Tortoise Plastron and Antler Horn Magic Syrup
Tortoise Shell and deer Antler Horn Combination
龟 鹿 二 仙 胶

■ Ingredients

Lu Jiao	Antler Horn	5000g
Gui Ban	Tortoise Palstron	2500g
Ren Shen	Ginseng	500g
Gou Qi Zi	Lycium Fruit	1500g

■ Preparation
Use as prepared form.

■ Pertaining Category
Yin Tonifying

■ Functions
Nourishes the kidney Yin and essence, warms the kidney Yang. Tonifies Qi and blood.

■ Indications
Deficiency of kidney Yin, Yang, and essence with insufficiency of Qi and blood manifested as pain and weakness of lower back and knees, emaciation, fatigue, impotence, nocturnal emission or spermatorrhea, dizziness, blurred vision, pale tongue with white coat, a deep, weak, and slow pulse.

■ Cautions and Contraindications
It is contraindicated in cases of exterior and heat patterns, Qi, blood, phlegm-dampness, and food stagnation.

■ Modern Applications
Chronic consumptive diseases, severe depletion due to prolonged illness, impotence, etc.

Gui Pi Tang-Restore the Spleen Decoction
Ginseng and Longan Combination
归 脾 汤

Ingredients

Bai Zhu	White Atractylodes	9g
Huang Qi	Astragalus	12g
Fu Ling	Hoelen/Poria	9-12g
Long Yan Rou	Longan	9g
Suan Zao Ren	Zizyphus	12g
Ren Shen	Ginseng	6g
Dang Gui	Chinese Angelica	6-9g
Yuan Zhi	Polygala	6g
Mu Xiang	Saussurea	6g
Sheng Jiang	Fresh Ginger	6g
Da Zao	Jujube	3-5pcs
Zhi Gan Cao	Baked Licorice	6g

■ Preparation

Use as decoction or prepared form.

■ Pertaining Category

Qi and Blood Tonifying

■ Functions

Tonifies Qi and blood, strengthens the spleen, nurishes the heart, calms spirit.

■ Indications

Deficiency of the spleen Qi and heart blood manifested as palpitation, insomnia, forgetfulness, poor appetite, lassitude, sallow complexion, shortened menstruation with excessive, thin, light colored flow, uterine bleeding, white clear vaginal discharge, pale tongue with thin white coat, a thin, weak pulse.

■ **Cautions and Contraindications**
It is contraindicated in cases of any excess or deficient heat patterns.

■ **Modern Applications**
Anemia, neurasthenia, peptic ulcer, chronic gastritis, functional uterine bleeding, irregular menstruation, chronic bleeding, vegetative (Autonomic) nerve dysfunction, cardiac neurosis, etc.

Gui Zhi Fu Ling Wan-Cinnamon Twig and Hoelen Pill
Cinnamon and Hoelen Formula
桂 枝 茯 苓 丸

■ **Ingredients**

Gui Zhi	Cinnamon Twig	9g
Fu Ling	Hoelen/Poria	9g
Mu Dan Pi	Moutan Bark	9g
Tao Ren	Peach Kernel	9g
Chi Shao Yao	Red Peony	9g

■ **Preparation**
Use as prepared form or decoction.

■ **Pertaining Category**
Blood Invigorating

■ **Functions**
Promotes blood circulation, removes blood stasis. Softens abdominal masses.

good for fibroids

■ Indications
Blood stasis and phlegm-dampness accumulating in the uterus manifested as lower abdominal masses with pain or discomfort, painful menstruation, or restless fetus with dark bleeding and abdominal pain aggravated by pressure, or retention of lochia with abdominal pain, purple tongue with greasy coat, a wiry, slippery, hesitant pulse.

■ Cautions and Contraindications
Use with extreme caution during pregnancy.

■ Modern Applications
Uterus fibroids, ovarian cyst, dysmenorrhea, endometriosis, retention of lochia, infertility, etc.

Gui Zhi Gan Cao Long Gu Mu Li Tang-Cinnamon, Licorice, Dragon Bone, and Oyster Shell Decoction
桂枝甘草龙骨牡蛎汤

■ Ingredients

Gui Zhi	Cinnamon Twig	3-6g
Zhi Gan Cao	Baked Licorice	6g
Long Gu	Dragon Bone	15g
Mu Li	Oyster Shell	15g

■ Preparation
Use as decoction or prepared form.

■ Pertaining Category
Additional Formulas for Internal Medicine

■ Functions
Warms the heart Yang, benefits the heart Yin. Calms spirit.

155

■ Indications

Taiyang disease or inappropriate using of warming herbs causing heart Yang and Yin deficiency manifested as palpitation, restlessness, a fullness sensation in the chest, shortness of breath, sweating, pale complexion, cold limbs, pale tongue with white coat, a deep, thin, weak, or intermittent pulse.

■ Cautions and Contraindications

None noted.

■ Modern Applications

Neurosis, neurasthenia, etc.

Gui Zhi Tang-Cinnamon Twig Decoction
Cinnamon Combination
桂 枝 汤

■ Ingredients

Gui Zhi	Cinnamon Twig	9g
Bai Shao Yao	White Peony	9g
Zhi Gan Cao	Baked Licorice	6g
Sheng Jiang	Fresh Ginger	9g
Da Zao	Jujube	3pcs

■ Preparation

Use as decoction or prepared form.

■ Pertaining Category

Pungent Warm Exterior Relieving

■ Functions

Promotes sweat, expels pathogen from the muscle layer, releases the exterior. Regulates nutritive Qi and defensive Qi.

■ Indications

Exterior deficiency with wind-cold invasion manifested as mild fever, headache, sweating, aversion to wind-cold, nasal congestion, retching, no thirst, thin white and moist tongue coat, a superficial, slow pulse.

■ Cautions and Contraindications

It is contraindicated in cases of exterior wind-heat, exterior wind-cold with internal heat.

■ Modern Applications

Common cold, influenza, upper respiratory tract infection, allergic rhinitis, abdominal pain, sciatica, skin diseases, urticaria, chilblain, etc.

Gun Tan Wan-Rolling Out Phlegm Pill
Lapis and Scute Formula
滚 痰 丸

■ Ingredients

Meng Shi	Lapis	30g
Da Huang	Rhubarb	240g
Huang Qin	Scute	240g
Chen Xiang	Aquilaria	15g

■ Preparation

Use as prepared form.

■ Pertaining Category

Heat Clearing and Phlegm Resolving

■ Functions

Purges fire, dispels phlegm.

■ Indications

Phlegm-fire disturbing the heart and orifices manifested as mania, severe palpitation, anxiety, insomnia, or coma, coughing and wheezing with yellow thick sputum, a fullness and stifling sensation in the chest and epigastrium, dizziness, tinnitus, or lumps in the neck, or constipation, red tongue with yellow thick greasy coat, a slippery, rapid, and forceful pulse.

■ Cautions and Contraindications

It is contraindicated during pregnancy and postpartum, or patients with weak constitution.

■ Modern Applications

Mania, hysteria, anxiety, neurosis, schizophrenia, seizures, acute infantile convulsion, bronchial asthma, acute bronchitis, chronic obstructive pulmonary disease, scrofula, etc.

Hai Zao Yu Hu Tang-Sargassum Jade Flask Decoction
The Seaweed Decoction
海藻玉壶汤

■ Ingredients

Hai Zao	Sargassum	3g
Kun Bu	Kelp Thallus	3g
Ban Xia	Pinellia Tuber	3g
Chen Pi	Tangerine Peel	3g
Qing Pi	Green Citrus Peel	3g
Lian Qiao	Forsythiaa Fruit	3g
Zhe Bei Mu	Thunberg Fritillary	3g
Dang Gui	Chinese Angelica	3g
Chuan Xiong	Ligusticum	3g
Du Huo	Tuhuo	3g
Hai Dai	Laminariae	1.5g
Gan Cao	Licorice	3g

■ Preparation
Use as decoction or prepared form.

■ Pertaining Category
Treating External Carbuncles

■ Functions
Resolves phlegm, softens hard lumps, reduces and disperses goiter.

■ Indications
Qi goiter due to disharmony between the liver and spleen with stagnation of phlegm, Qi, and blood manifested as hard, painless, and immobile lumps on the neck without color change of skin, a fullness sensation in the chest and hypochondriac region, thin, greasy tongue coat, a wiry, slippery pulse.

■ Cautions and Contraindications
None noted.

■ Modern Applications
Goiter, hyperthyroidism, benign tumors of the thyroid, lymphadenitis, etc.

Hao Qin Qing Dan Tang-Sweet Wormwood and Scute Decoction to Clear the Gallbladder
Sweet Wormwood and Scute Combination
蒿 芩 清 胆 汤

■ Ingredients

Qing Hao	Sweet Wormwood	6g
Huang Qin	Scute	6g
Ban Xia	Pinellia Tuber	5g
Zhu Ru	Bamboo Shavings	9g
Chi Fu Ling	Red Poria	9g
Zhi Ke	Bitter Orange	5g
Chen Pi	Tangerine Peel	5g
Hua Shi	Talcum	6g
Gan Cao	Licorice	1.5g
Qing Dai	Indigo	1.5g

■ Preparation

Use as decoction, place last three ingredients (powder) in the cheese cloth bag, cook it with other ingredients; or use as prepared form.

■ Pertaining Category

Shaoyang Harmonizing (Mediating)

■ Functions

Clears damp-heat in the gallbladder, resolves phlegm, harmonizes the stomach.

■ Indications

Damp-heat affecting the gallbladder and Shaoyang channel manifested as alternate mild chills and pronounced fever, a stifling sensation in the chest, a bitter taste in the mouth, dry throat, bitter or sour fluids regurgitation, or vomiting of yellow-sticky fluids, or dry heaves in severe case, distending pain in the chest and hypochondrium, dark and scanty urine, red tongue with white or yellow greasy coat, a wiry, slippery, and rapid pulse.

■ Cautions and Contraindications

None noted.

■ Modern Applications

Acute cholecystitis, acute hepatitis, acute gastroenteritis, acute or chronic pancreatitis, malaria, etc.

He Che Da Zao Wan-Human Placenta Major Tonifying Pill

Pills of Human Placenta

河车大造丸

■ Ingredients

Zi He Che	Human Placenta	3g
Shu Di Huang	Cooked Rehmannia	6g
Du Zhong	Eucommia Bark	4.5g
Tian Men Dong	Asparagus	3g
Mai Men Dong	Ophiopogon	3g
Gui Ban	Tortoise Plastron	6g
Huang Bai	Phellodendron	4.5g
Niu Xi	Achyranthes	3g

■ Preparation
Use as decoction or prepared form.

■ Pertaining Category
Yin Tonifying

■ Functions
Nourishes Yin, replenishes the kidney essence. Subdues deficient fire.

■ Indications
Lung, liver, and kidney Yin deficiency with insufficiency of kidney essence and deficient fire manifested as soreness and weakness of lower back, dizziness, tinnitus, retarded mental and physical development in children, tidal fever, cough with scanty blood tinged sputum, or weight loss, red tongue with no coat or slight thin yellow coat, a thin, weak, rapid pulse.

- ■ **Cautions and Contraindications**

None noted.

- ■ **Modern Applications**

Chronic lower back pain, chronic nephritis, tinnitus, pulmonary tuberculosis, retarded development in children, etc.

He Ren Yin-Fleece Flower and Ginseng Beverage
Fleece Flower and Ginseng Combination
何人饮

- ■ **Ingredients**

He Shou Wu	Fleece Flower Root	9-20g
Ren Shen	Ginseng	9-12g
Dang Gui	Chinese Angelica	6-9g
Chen Pi	Tangerine Peel	6-9g
Wei Jiang	Roasted Ginger	6-9g

- ■ **Preparation**

Use as decoction or prepared form.

- ■ **Pertaining Category**

Additional Formulas for Internal Medicine

- ■ **Functions**

Nourishes blood, tonifies Qi, treats malarial disorders.

- ■ **Indications**

Chronic malaria with the liver blood and spleen Qi deficiency manifested as alternate chills and fever that is aggravated by only slight amount of exertion, sallow complexion, emaciation, poor appetite, lassitude, shortness of breath, dislike to speak, pale tongue, a thin, weak pulse.

■ **Cautions and Contraindications**

It is contraindicated during the early stage of a malaria and in cases without deficiency.

■ **Modern Applications**

Malarial disorders, etc.

Hou Po Wen Zhong Tang-Magnolia Bark Decoction to Warm the Middle Burner
Magnolia and Saussurea Combination
厚朴温中汤

■ **Ingredients**

Hou Po	Magnolia Bark	9-15g
Chen Pi	Tangerine Peel	9-15g
Fu Ling	Hoelen/Poria	9-12g
Cao Dou Kou	Alpinia	6-9g
Mu Xiang	Saussurea	6-9g
Gan Jiang	Dried Ginger	2-6g
Zhi Gan Cao	Baked Licorice	3-6g
Sheng Jiang	Fresh Ginger	3slices

■ **Preparation**

Use as decoction or prepared form.

■ **Pertaining Category**

Qi Regulating (Moving)

■ **Functions**

Warms the middle burner, dispels cold. Moves Qi, dries dampness, relieves abdominal distention.

Indications

Damp-cold obstructing Qi in the middle burner manifested as distention and pain in the epigastrium and abdomen, poor appetite, lassitude, loose stools, or vomiting of clear fluid, white and moist tongue coat, a slippery pulse.

Cautions and Contraindications

None noted.

Modern Applications

Chronic gastroenteritis, intestinal adhesion, peptic ulcer, chronic pancreatitis, indigestion, inflammatory bowel syndrome, etc.

Hu Qian Wan-The Hidden Tiger Pill
Tiger Bone and Tortoise Shell Formula
虎潜丸

Ingredients

Huang Bai	*Phellodendron*	150g
Gui Ban	*Tortoise Plastron*	120g
Zhi Mu	*Anemarrhena*	60g
Shu Di Huang	*Cooked Rehmannia*	60g
Chen Pi	*Tangerine Peel*	60g
Bai Shao Yao	*White Peony*	60g
Suo Yang	*Cynomorium*	45g
Hu Gu	*Tiger Bone*	30g
Gan Jiang	*Dried Ginger*	15g

Preparation

Use as prepared form or decoction with properly reduced dosage.

Pertaining Category

Yin Tonifying

■ Functions

Nourishes the kidney Yin, reduces deficient fire. Strengthens the bones and sinews.

■ Indications

Yin deficiency of the liver and kidney with deficient fire and weakness of bones and tendons manifested as soreness and weakness of lower back, flaccidity and atrophy of lower limbs, joint swelling and deformities, walking difficulty, red tongue with scanty coat, a thin, weak pulse.

■ Cautions and Contraindications

It is contraindicated in cases of atrophy due to deficiency of the spleen and stomach or damp-heat,

■ Modern Applications

Sequelae of polio, bone tuberculosis, fracture of lower limbs, elderly osteoarthritis, especially in the lower limbs, osteoporosis, etc.

Hua Gai San-Canopy Powder
Ma Huang and Morus Formula
华 盖 散

■ Ingredients

Ma Huang	Ephedra	30g
Sang Bai Pi	Morus Rootbark	30g
Zi Su Zi	Perilla Seed	30g
Xing Ren	Apricot Seed	30g
Chi Fu Ling	Sclerotium Poria	30g
Chen Pi	Tangerine Peel	30g
Zhi Gan Cao	Baked licorice	15g

■ Preparation

Use as prepared form or decoction with properly reduced dosage.

■   **Pertaining Category**
Pungent Warm Exterior Relieving

■   **Functions**
Disperses the lung Qi, releases the exterior. Resolves phlegm, stops coughing.

■   **Indications**
Wind-cold affecting the lungs with retention of phlegm manifested as cough with copious sputum, a fullness sensation in the chest, difficulty in breathing, thin white tongue coat, a superficial pulse.

■   **Cautions and Contraindications**
It is contraindicated in cases of exterior deficiency. Use with caution for patients with hypertension and heart problems.

■   **Modern Applications**
Common cold, influenza, upper respiratory tract infection, bronchitis bronchial asthma, pneumonia, whooping cough, etc.

Huai Hua San-Sophora Japonica Flower Powder
Sophora Flower Formula
槐 花 散

■   **Ingredients**

Huai Hua	Sophora Flower	12g
Ce Bai Ye	Biota Leaves	12g
Jing Jie Sui	Schizonepeta Spike	6g
Zhi Ke	Bitter Orange	6g

■   **Preparation**
Use as decoction or prepared form.

■   **Pertaining Category**
Stopping Bleeding

166

Functions
Clears toxic heat in the intestines, stops bleeding. Dispels wind, descends the adverse flow of Qi.

Indications
Wind-heat invasion or damp-heat leading to intestinal wind and toxic-heat damaging blood vessels manifested as rectal bleeding before or after passing stools or with stools, or internal hemorrhoids fresh red blood or dull purplish blood, red tongue with yellow coat, a wiry, rapid pulse.

Cautions and Contraindications
Do not use this formula for long term. It is contraindicated in cases of bloody stools without damp-heat.

Modern Applications
Hemorrhoids, ulcerative colitis, proctopolypus, amebic dysentery, anal fissure, etc.

Huai Jiao Wan-Sophora Japonica Fruit Pill
Sophora Fruit Pill
槐 角 丸

Ingredients

Huai Jiao	Pagoda Tree Fruit	500g
Fang Feng	Siler	250g
Di Yu	Sanguisorba	250g
Dang Gui	Chinese Angelica	250g
Huang Qin	Scute	250g
Zhi Ke	Bitter Orange	250g

Preparation
Use as prepared form or decoction with properly reduced dosage.

Pertaining Category
Stopping Bleeding

Functions

Clears heat in the intestines, stops bleeding. Dispels wind, regulates Qi.

Indications

Toxic wind-heat invasion or damp-heat accumulating in the intestines manifested as bloody stools, hemorrhoids, prolapse of anus, constipation, red tongue with thin yellow greasy coat, a rapid pulse.

Cautions and Contraindications

None noted.

Modern Applications

Hemorrhoids, etc.

Huang Lian E Jiao Tang-Coptis and Donkey-hide Gelatin Decoction

Coptis and Donkey-hide Combination

黄 连 阿 胶 汤

Ingredients

Huang Lian	Coptis	12g
Huang Qin	Scute	6g
E Jiao	Equus/Gelatin	9g
Bai Shao Yao	White Peony	6g
Ji Zi Huang	Egg Yolk	2pcs

Preparation

Use as decoction or prepared form. E Jiao should be dissolved separately in boiling water and added into the strained decoction. Egg Yolks are boiled hard and mixed into the strained decoction.

Pertaining Category

Yin Tonifying

■ **Functions**

Nourishes Yin, descends fire, relieves irritability, calms spirit.

■ **Indications**

Yin deficiency of the heart and kidney with heart fire or later stage of febrile disease affecting the spirit manifested as a irritable heat and stifling sensation in the chest, palpitation, anxiety, insomnia, dry mouth and throat, red tongue with dry, yellow coat, a deep, thin and rapid pulse.

■ **Cautions and Contraindications**

None noted.

■ **Modern Applications**

Neurasthenia, insomnia, etc.

Huang Lian Jie Du Tang-Coptis Relieve Toxicity Decoction
Coptis and Scute Combination
黄连解毒汤

■ **Ingredients**

Huang Lian	Coptis	9g
Huang Qin	Scute	6g
Huang Bai	Phellodendron	6g
Zhi Zi	Gardenia Fruit	9g

■ **Preparation**

Use as decoction or prepared form.

■ **Pertaining Category**

Heat Clearing and Detoxicating

■ **Functions**

Drains fire-heat from all three burners, relieves toxicity.

■ Indications

Toxic heat or damp heat in three burners manifested as high fever, irritability, insomnia or delirium, dry mouth and throat, vomiting of blood, nosebleeding, or skin rashes, dysenteric disorder, jaundice, carbuncles, deep-rooted boils or toxic swellings, scanty and yellow urine, red tongue with yellow coat, a rapid, forceful pulse.

■ Cautions and Contraindications

It is contraindicated in cases of the spleen and stomach Yang deficiency or Yin deficiency with deep-red and uncoated tongue.

■ Modern Applications

Influenza, encephalitis B, meningitis, septicemia, pyogenic skin infection, hepatitis, acute gastroenteritis or dysentery, acute UTI, acute cholecystitis, as well as stomatitis, toothache, and laryngopharyngitis, etc.

Huang Lian Tang-Coptis Decoction
Coptis Combination
黄 连 汤

■ Ingredients

Huang Lian	Coptis	5g
Gan Jiang	Dried Ginger	5g
Gui Zhi	Cinnamon Twig	5g
Ren Shen	Ginseng	3g
Ban Xia	Pinellia Tuber	9g
Zhi Gan Cao	Baked Licorice	6g
Da Zao	Jujube	4pcs

■ Preparation

Use as decoction or prepared form.

■ Pertaining Category

Regulating the Intestines and Stomach (Mediating)

■ **Functions**

Regulates cold and heat, harmonizes the stomach, descends rebellious stomach Qi downward.

■ **Indications**

Upper burner heat with middle burner cold manifested as a stifling sensation in the chest, irritability, nausea or vomiting, abdominal pain, borborygmus, diarrhea, red tip or pale tongue with white greasy coat, a wiry, slippery pulse.

■ **Cautions and Contraindications**

It is contraindicated in cases of retching and nausea due to stomach Yin deficiency.

■ **Modern Applications**

Acute or chronic gastroenteritis, peptic ulcer, indigestion, gastrointestinal neurosis, morning sickness, etc.
This formula is modified from Ban Xia Xie Xin Tang (Pinellia Decoction to Purge the Stomach).

Huang Long Tang-Yellow Dragon Decoction
Ginseng and Rhubarb Combination
黄 龙 汤

■ **Ingredients**

Da Huang	Rhubarb	12g
Mang Xiao	Mirabilitum	9g
Zhi Shi	Immature Citrus	9g
Hou Po	Magnolia Bark	12g
Ren Shen	Ginseng	6g
Dang Gui	Chinese Angelica	9g
Gan Cao	Licorice	3g
Jie Geng	Platycodon	3g
Sheng Jiang	Fresh Ginger	3 slices
Da Zao	Jujube	2pcs

■ **Preparation**

Use as decoction or prepared form. Mang Xiao (Mirabilitum) should be infused in the strained decoction.

■ **Pertaining Category**

Purging Downward with Tonifying Effect

■ **Functions**

Purges heat downward, promotes bowel movement. Tonifies Qi and blood.

■ **Indications**

Interior heat accumulation with Qi and blood deficiency manifested as watery foul-smelling diarrhea, or constipation, epigastric fullness, abdominal distention and pain which is worse with pressure, fever, thirst, or delirium, dry mouth and tongue, fatigue, shortness of breath, dry yellow or black coat,a weak pulse.

■ **Cautions and Contraindications**

It is contraindicated during pregnancy.

■ **Modern Applications**

Intestinal obstruction, elderly, postpartum, or habitual constipation, epidemic or non-epidemic febrile diseases, etc.

This formula has similar effects as Xin Jia Huang Long Tang (Newly Augmented Yellow Dragon Decoction), but this formula has stronger effect of purging downward, while has weaker tonifying effect.

Huang Qi Gui Zhi Wu Wu Tang-Astragalus and Cinnamon Twig Five Substances Decoction
Astragalus and Cinnamon Five Herbs Combination
黄芪桂枝五物汤

■ Ingredients

Huang Qi	Astragalus	12g
Gui Zhi	Cinnamon Twig	9g
Bai Shao Yao	White Peony	9g
Sheng Jiang	Fresh Ginger	12g
Da Zao	Jujube	4pcs

■ Preparation
Use as decoction or prepared form.

■ Pertaining Category
Channel Warming and Cold Dispelling

■ Functions
Tonifies Qi, warms the channels, dispels cold, harmonizes blood circulation, relieves pain.

■ Indications
Blood stagnation in the channels with Qi deficiency and mild wind invasion manifested as numbness of the body and limbs, arthralgia with mild pain, intolerance to wind, pale tongue with white coat, a slight tight, and hesitant pulse.

■ Cautions and Contraindications
None noted.

■ Modern Applications
Arthritis, mild neuralgia, etc.

Huang Qi Jian Zhong Tang-Astragalus Strengthen the Middle Burner Decoction
Astragalus Combination
黄 芪 建 中 汤

■ Ingredients

Huang Qi	Astragalus	9g
Gui Zhi	Cinnamon Twig	9g
Bai Shao Yao	White Peony	18g
Zhi Gan Cao	Baked Licorice	6g
Sheng Jiang	Fresh Ginger	9g
Da Zao	Jujube	12pcs
Yi Tang	Maltose	18-30g

■ Preparation
Use as decoction or prepared form.

■ Pertaining Category
Middle Burner Warming and Cold Dispelling

■ Functions
Warms and tonifies the spleen and stomach Qi. Harmonizes middle burner, relieves spasmodic abdominal pain.

■ Indications
Chronic consumptive disease with severe deficiency Qi of the spleen and stomach and interior spasm in the middle burner manifested as prolonged intermittent, spasmodic abdominal pain which can be alleviated by local warmth and pressure, pale complexion, poor appetite, fatigue, palpitation, cold limbs, shortness of breath, pale tongue with white coat, a thin weak pulse.

■ Cautions and Contraindications
It is contraindicated in cases of vomiting, round worms, abdominal distention, and heat from Yin deficiency.

■ Modern Applications
Peptic ulcer, neurasthenia, aplastic anemia, chronic gastroenteritis, chronic hepatitis, gastric and intestinal spasms, chronic appendicitis, etc.

This formula is modified from Xiao Jian Zhong Tang (Minor Strengthen the Middle Burner Decoction).

174

Huang Qi Tang-Astragalus Decoction
Astragalus Combination
黄芪汤

■ **Ingredients**

Huang Qi	Astragalus	30g
Chen Pi	Tangerine Peel	9g
Huo Ma Ren	Hemp Seed	15g
Feng Mi	Honey	15g

■ **Preparation**
Use as decoction or prepared form. Honey should be stirred into the strained decoction.

■ **Pertaining Category**
Additional Formulas for Internal Medicine

■ **Functions**
Tonifies Qi, moistens the intestines, relaxes bowel movement.

■ **Indications**
Constipation due to Qi deficiency manifested as difficulty in eliminating the bowels even though patient has the urge, the stools are neither too hard nor dry, no abdominal distention and pain, pale complexion, shortness of breath, spontaneous sweating, fatigue, pale and delicate tongue with thin white coat, a weak pulse.

■ **Cautions and Contraindications**
It is contraindicated in cases of constipation due to excess.

■ **Modern Applications**
Constipation in elderly, weak constitution, and post-surgery, etc.

Huang Qin Tang-Scute Decoction
Scute and Licorice Combination
黄芩汤

■ **Ingredients**

Huang Qin	Scute	9g
Bai Shao Yao	White Peony	9g
Zhi Gan Cao	Baked Licorice	3g
Da Zao	Jujube	4pcs

■ **Preparation**

Use as decoction or prepared form.

■ **Pertaining Category**

Clearing Heat from Zang-fu Organs

■ **Functions**

Clears heat, relieves dysentery and diarrhea. Harmonizes middle burner, alleviates pain.

■ **Indications**

Heat entering the intestines manifested as fever, a bitter taste in the mouth, diarrhea, dysentery, abdominal pain, red tongue with yellow coat, a rapid pulse.

■ **Cautions and Contraindications**

None noted.

■ **Modern Applications**

Enteritis, dysentery, etc.

Huang Tu Tang-Baked Yellow Earth Decoction

Fu-lung-kan Combination
黄土汤

■ Ingredients

Zao Xin Huang Tu	Baked Yellow Earth	18-30g
Bai Zhu	White Atractylodes	9g
Fu Zi	Prepared Aconite	9g
Sheng Di Huang	Dried Rehmannia	9g
E Jiao	Equus/Gelatin	9g
Huang Qin	Scute	9g
Gan Cao	Licorice	9g

■ Preparation
Decoct the Baked Yellow Earth in water separately for 30 minutes to get its decoction, then decoct other herbs in the decoction. E Jiao should be dissolved separately in boiling water, then added into the strained decoction.

■ Pertaining Category
Stopping Bleeding

■ Functions
Warms the spleen Yang, tonifies the spleen Qi. Nourishes blood, stops bleeding.

■ Indications
Deficiency of the spleen Yang and Qi with inability to control blood manifested as bloody or dark stools, uterine bleeding, vomiting of blood, nosebleeding, pale or dark red blood, cold limbs, sallow complexion, pale tongue with white coat, a deep, thin, and weak pulse.

■ **Cautions and Contraindications**
It is contraindicated in cases of bleeding with existing exterior patterns.

■ **Modern Applications**
Chronic hemorrhage of digestive tract such as peptic ulcer, chronic functional uterine bleeding, etc.

Huo Luo Xiao Ling Dan-Effectively Invigorate the Collaterals Elixir
Salvia and Tang-kuei Combination
活 络 效 灵 丹

■ **Ingredients**

Dan Shen	Salvia Root	15g
Dang Gui	Chinese Angelica	15g
Ru Xiang	Frankincense	15g
Mo Yao	Myrrh	15g

■ **Preparation**
Use as prepared form or decoction with properly reduced dosage.

■ **Pertaining Category**
Blood Invigorating

■ **Functions**
Invigorates blood, removes blood stasis. Unblocks channels and collaterals, stops pain.

■ **Indications**
Internal or external blood stasis due to Qi stagnation or trauma manifested as pain in the chest, epigastrium, abdomen, back, or limbs, swelling and bruising, internal and external ulcerations, fixed abdominal masses, or rheumatic pain, purple tongue, a wiry, hesitant pulse.

178

Cautions and Contraindications
It is contraindicated during pregnancy or any bleeding disorders.

Modern Applications
Angina pectoris, cerebral thrombosis, ectopic pregnancy, traumatic injury, arthritis, sciatica, pelvic inflammatory disease, etc.

Huo Po Xia Ling Tang-Agastache, Magnolia, Pinellia, and Poria Decoction
Agastache and Magnolia Combination
藿朴夏苓汤

Ingredients

Huo Xiang	*Agastache*	6g
Hou Po	*Magnolia Bark*	3g
Ban Xia	*Pinellia Tuber*	4.5g
Chi Fu Ling	*Hoelen/Poria*	9g
Zhu Ling	*Polyporus*	4.5g
Xing Ren	*Apricot Seed*	9g
Yi Yi Ren	*Coix Seed*	12g
Bai Dou Kou	*Cluster Fruit*	2g
Ze Xie	*Alisma Tuber*	4.5g
Dan Dou Chi	*Prepared Soybean*	9g

Preparation
Use as decoction or prepared form.

Pertaining Category
Damp-heat Clearing

Functions
Expels wind-damp-heat, releases the exterior. Transforms dampness.

179

■ **Indications**

Wind-damp-heat invasion with internal dampness retention manifested as chills, fever, heaviness of body and limbs, lassitude, stifling sensation in the chest, stickiness of mouth, white, thin, greasy tongue coat, a slippery, soft, and slow pulse.

■ **Cautions and Contraindications**

It is contraindicated in cases of deficiency of Yin, blood, and body fluids.

■ **Modern Applications**

Acute gastroenteritis, influenza, acute hepatitis, acute pyelonephritis, etc.

Huo Xiang Zheng Qi San-Agastache Qi Rectifying Powder
Agastache Formula
藿 香 正 气 散

■ **Ingredients**

Huo Xiang	Agastache	90g
Ban Xia	Pinellia Tuber	60g
Bai Zhu	White Atractylodes	60g
Chen Pi	Tangerine Peel	60g
Hou Po	Magnolia Bark	60g
Jie Geng	Platycodon	60g
Da Fu Pi	Areca Peel	30g
Bai Zhi	Angelica Root	30g
Zi Su Ye	Perilla Leaf	30g
Fu Ling	Hoelen/Poria	30g
Zhi Gan Cao	Baked Licorice	75g
Sheng Jiang	Fresh Ginger	3slices
Da Zao	Jujube	1pc

■ **Preparation**

Use as prepared form or decoction with properly reduced dosage.
Do not decoct for more than 20 minutes.

■ **Pertaining Category**

Dampness Drying and Stomach Harmonizing

■ **Functions**

Expels wind-cold, releases the exterior. Transforms turbid
dampness, moves Qi, harmonizes the middle burner.

■ **Indications**

External wind-cold with internal dampness obstructing Qi in the
middle burner manifested as chills, fever, headache, fullness in the
chest, epigastric and abdominal distention and pain, nausea,
vomiting, borborygmus, diarrhea, white, thick, and greasy tongue
coat, a superficial, tight, or slippery pulse.

■ **Cautions and Contraindications**

It is contraindicated in cases of Yin deficiency with empty fire.
Use with extreme caution for patients with thirst and yellow
tongue coat.

■ **Modern Applications**

Influenza, common cold of gastrointestinal type, acute
gastroenteritis, peptic ulcer, colitis, food poisoning, etc.

Ji Chuan Jian-Benefit the River Decoction
Tangkuei and Cistanche Combination
济 川 煎

■ **Ingredients**

Dang Gui	Chinese Angelica	9-15g
Rou Cong Rong	Cistanche	6-9g
Huai Niu Xi	Achyranthes	6g
Ze Xie	Alisma	4.5g
Sheng Ma	Cimicifuga	1.5-3g
Zhi Ke	Bitter Orange	3g

■ **Preparation**

Use as decoction or prepared form.

■ **Pertaining Category**

Purging Downward with Moist Laxatives

■ **Functions**

Warms the kidneys, replenishes blood and essence. Moistens the intestines, promotes bowel movement.

■ **Indications**

Constipation due to kidney Yang and essence deficiency accompanied by clear and copious urine, soreness of lower back and knees with a cold sensation, dizziness, especially in elderly person, pale tongue with thin white coat, a thin, weak pulse.

■ **Cautions and Contraindications**

It is contraindicated in cases of constipation due to excess heat.

■ **Modern Applications**

Habitual constipation, anemia, postpartum, and elderly person with constipation and osteoarthritis.

Ji Jiao Li Huang Wan-Stephania, Zanthoxylum, Lepidium, and Rhubarb Pill
Stephania and Lepidium Formula
己 椒 苈 黄 丸

■ **Ingredients**

Fang Ji	Stephania Root	12g
Hua Jiao	Zanthoxylum	4.5g
Ting Li Zi	Lepidium Seed	9g
Da Huang	Rhubarb	9g

■ **Preparation**
Use as decoction or prepared form.

■ **Pertaining Category**
Additional Formulas for Internal Medicine

■ **Functions**
Drains water and congested fluid, reduces edema. Purges heat, moves bowels.

■ **Indications**
Accumulated water and heat obstructing Qi in the stomach and large intestine manifested as edema with dyspnea, abdominal distention, constipation, borborygmus, dry mouth, red tongue with yellow greasy coat, a slippery, deep, and rapid pulse.

■ **Cautions and Contraindications**
It is contraindicated during pregnancy and for patients with weak constitution. Do not use overdose and for long term.

■ **Modern Applications**
Ascites from liver cirrhosis, edema from chronic pulmonary heart disease, or ascariasis, etc.

Ji Ming San-Powder to Take at Cock's Crow
Areca Seed and Chaenomeles Formula
鸡鸣散

Ingredients

Bing Lang	Betel Nut	15g
Chen Pi	Tagerine Peel	9g
Mu Gua	Chaenomeles Fruit	9g
Wu Zhu Yu	Evodia	3g
Zi Su Ye	Perilla Leaf	3g
Jie Geng	Platycodon	5g
Sheng Jiang	Fresh Ginger	5g

■ Preparation
Use as decoction or prepared form.

■ Pertaining Category
Wind-dampness Expelling

■ Functions
Transforms cold-damp, descends the turbidity, moves Qi.

■ Indications
Cold-damp obstructing in the channels of lower limbs manifested as cold pain and swollen in the legs with heaviness and numbness, or spasms of muscles, difficulty in walking, chills or fever, a fullness sensation in the chest, nausea, pale tongue with white greasy coat, a slow, soft pulse.

■ Cautions and Contraindications
It should not be used in cases of leg Qi due to damp-heat without modification.

■ Modern Applications
Beriberi, edema, filariasis, etc.

Ji Sheng Shen Qi Wan-Kidney Qi Pill for Aiding the Living
Rehmannia Eight Formula Plus Cyathula and Palntago

济生肾气丸

■ **Ingredients**

Shu Di Huang	Cooked Rehmannia	15g
Shan Zhu Yu	Dogwood Fruit	30g
Shan Yao	Dioscorea	30g
Ze Xie	Alisma	30g
Fu Ling	Hoelen/Poria	30g
Mu Dan Pi	Moutan Bark	30g
Fu Zi	Prepared Aconite	15g
Rou Gui	Cinnamon Bark	15g
Chuan Niu Xi	Cyathula	15g
Che Qian Zi	Plantago	30g

■ **Preparation**

Use as prepared form or decoction with properly reduced dosage.
Che Qian Zi should be wrapped in gauze when making decoction.

■ **Pertaining Category**

Yang Tonifying

■ **Functions**

Warms the kidney Yang, tonifies the kidney Qi. Promotes urination,
reduces edema.

■ **Indications**

Deficiency of the kidney Yang and Qi with water retention
manifested as edema below the waist with heavy sensation, soreness
of lower back, scanty, difficult urination, aversion to cold, cold
limbs, abdominal distention, pale and swollen tongue with tooth
marks and white moist coat, a deep, thin, slippery, or wiry pulse.

■ **Cautions and Contraindications**
It is contraindicated in cases of deficient fire due to Yin deficiency,
consumption of body fluid from dry heat.

■ **Modern Applications**
Edema from chronic nephritis, hypothyroidism, pulmonary
emphysema, pulmonary heart disease, chronic bronchitis or asthma,
etc.

Jia Jian Fu Mai Tang-Modified Decoction for Restoring the Pulse
Modified Baked Licorice Decoction
加减复脉汤

■ **Ingredients**

Zhi Gan Cao	Baked Licorice	6-9g
Sheng Di Huang	Dried Rehmannia	15g
Bai Shao Yao	White Peony	12g
Mai Men Dong	Ophiopogon	9-12g
E Jiao	Equus/Gelatin	9g
Huo Ma Ren	Hemp Seed	9g

■ **Preparation**
Use as decoction or prepared form. E Jiao should be dissolved
separately in boiling water and added into the strained decoction.

■ **Pertaining Category**
Yin Tonifying

■ **Functions**
Nourishes Yin and blood, generates body fluids, moistens dryness.

186

■ Indications

Deficiency of Yin and blood with dry heat manifested as chronic lower fever, a feverish sensation in the palms and soles, red face, dry mouth and throat, palpitation, restlessness, dry stools, red and dry tongue with no coat, a large and forceless pulse.

■ Cautions and Contraindications

It is contraindicated in cases of diarrhea due to deficiency of the spleen and stomach.

■ Modern Applications

Later stage of febrile diseases, constipation, hyperthyroidism, neurasthenia, chronic consumptive diseases, etc.

Jia Jian Wei Rui Tang-Modified
Polygonatum Decoction
Polygonatum and Mentha Combination
加减葳蕤汤

■ Ingredients

Wei Rui (Yu Zhu)	*Polygonatum*	9g
Bai Wei	*Swallowwort*	3g
Cong Bai	*Allium Bulb*	6g
Dan Dou Chi	*Prepared Soybean*	9g
Jie Geng	*Platycodon*	5g
Bo He	*Peppermint*	5g
Da Zao	*Jujube*	2pcs
Zhi Gan Cao	*Baked Licorice*	2g

■ Preparation

Use as decoction or prepared form.

■ Pertaining Category

Strengthening Body Resistance and Relieving Exterior

■ **Functions**

Nourishes Yin, clears heat. Promotes sweat, disperses wind-heat, releases the exterior.

■ **Indications**

Invasion of wind-heat with Yin deficiency constitution manifested as fever, slight aversion to cold without sweating or lack of sweating, headache, thirst, dry throat, irritability, or cough with sputum that is hard to expectorate, red tongue, a rapid pulse.

■ **Cautions and Contraindications**

It is contraindicated in cases of exterior pattern without Yin deficiency.

■ **Modern Applications**

Common cold, influenza, bronchitis, etc.

Jia Wei Xiang Su San-Augmented Cyperus and Perilla Leaf Powder

Cyperus, Perilla, and Siler Formula
加味香苏散

■ **Ingredients**

Zi Su Ye	Perilla Leaf	5g
Xiang Fu	Cyperus	4g
Chen Pi	Tangerine Peel	4g
Jing Jie	Schizonepeta	3g
Qin Jiao	Big Leaf Gentiana	3g
Fang Feng	Siler	3g
Man Jing Zi	Vitex Fruit	3g
Chuan Xiong	Ligusticum	1.5g
Sheng Jiang	Fresh Ginger	3slices
Zhi Gan Cao	Baked Licorice	2.5g

■ **Preparation**
Use as decoction or prepared form.

■ **Pertaining Category**
Pungent Warm Exterior Relieving

■ **Functions**
Promotes sweat, expels wind-cold, releases the exterior. Regulates Qi, stops pain.

■ **Indications**
Invasion of wind-cold with Qi stagnation manifested as aversion to wind-cold, fever, headache, neck stiffness, nasal congestion or running clear mucus, body aches, lack of sweat, a fullness sensation in the chest and epigastrium, belching, poor appetite, thin white tongue coat, a superficial pulse.

■ **Cautions and Contraindications**
None noted.

■ **Modern Applications**
Common cold, influenza, headache, sinus, etc.

Jia Wei Xiao Yao San-Augmented Wandering Powder
Bupleurum and Peony Combination
加 味 逍 遙 散

■ **Ingredients**

Chai Hu	Bupleurum	9g
Dang Gui	Chinese Angelica	9g
Bai Shao Yao	White Peony	12g
Bai Zhu	White Atractylodes	9g
Fu Ling	Hoelen/Poria	15g
Bo He	Peppermint	3g
Wei Jiang	Roasted Ginger	6g
Zhi Gan Cao	Baked Licorice	6g
Mu Dan Pi	Moutan Bark	6-9g
Zhi Zi	Gardenia Fruit	3-6g

■ **Preparation**
Use as decoction or prepared form.

■ **Pertaining Category**
Regulating the Liver and Spleen (Mediating)

■ **Functions**
Disperses liver Qi, relieves stagnation. Clears heat. Tonifies the spleen Qi. Harmonizes blood, regulates menstruation.

■ Indications

Liver and spleen disharmony with heat manifested as irritability, angry easily, headache, red or blood-shot eyes, irregular menstruation, lower abdominal pain with heavy sensation, painful and scanty urination, red cheek, dry mouth, spontaneous or night sweats, light purple and red sides tongue with thin white or yellow coat, a wiry, rapid pulse.

■ Cautions and Contraindications

None noted.

■ Modern Applications

Chronic hepatitis, peptic ulcer, irregular menstruation, uterine bleeding, premenstrual syndrome, menopausal syndrome, mental depression, hysteria, etc.

This formula is also known as Dan Zhi Xiao Yao San and is modified from Xiao Yao San (Wandering Powder).

Jian Pi Wan-Strengthen the Spleen Pill

Pill for Invigorating the Spleen

健 脾 丸

■ Ingredients

Bai Zhu	White Atractylodes	75g
Mu Xiang	Saussurea	22.5g
Huang Lian	Coptis	22.5g
Fu Ling	Hoelen/Poria	60g
Ren Shen	Ginseng	45g
Shen Qu	Medicated Leaven	30g
Chen Pi	Tangerine Peel	30g
Sha Ren	Amomum Fruit	30g
Mai Ya	Barley Sprout	30g
Shan Zha	Crataegus Fruit	30g
Shan Yao	Dioscorea	30g
Rou Dou Kou	Nutmeg	30g
Gan Cao	Licorice	22.5g

■ Preparation
Use as prepared form or decoction with properly reduced dosage.

■ Pertaining Category
Food Stagnation Relieving

■ Functions
Tonifies the spleen, harmonizes the stomach. Relieves food stagnation, stops diarrhea.

■ Indications
Severe spleen and stomach Qi deficiency with food stagnation manifested as poor appetite, indigestion, a stuffiness sensation in the epigastrium, abdominal distention, diarrhea, pale tongue with white or yellowish greasy coat, a weak, soft pulse.

■ **Cautions and Contraindications**

It is contraindicated in cases of acute food stagnation due to improper eating, overeating, or overdrinking.

■ **Modern Applications**

Chronic enteritis, ulcerative colitis, intestinal dysfunction, indigestion, irritable bowel syndrome, chronic gastritis, peptic ulcer, chronic dysentery, gastric prolapse, Crohn's disease, etc.

Jiao Ai Tang-Donkey-hide Gelatin and Mugwort Leaf Decoction
Tang-kuei and Equus Combination
胶艾汤

■ **Ingredients**

E Jiao	*Equus/Gelatin*	6-9g
Ai Ye	*Mugwort Leaf*	9g
Chuan Xiong	*Ligusticum*	6g
Dang Gui	*Chinese Angelica*	9g
Bai Shao Yao	*White Peony*	12g
Sheng Di Huang	*Dried Rehmannia*	12-18g
Gan Cao	*Licorice*	6g

■ **Preparation**

Use as decoction or prepared form. E Jiao should be dissolved separately in boiling water and added into strained decoction.

■ **Pertaining Category**

Stopping Bleeding

■ **Functions**

Nourishes blood, stops bleeding. Regulates menses, calms fetus.

■ **Indications**

Imbalance of the Chong and Ren channels with Yin blood deficiency manifested as excessive menstruation or uterine bleeding, or postpartum bleeding, or bleeding during pregnancy with abdominal pain, the blood is pale and thin quality without clots, pale tongue, a slow, thin, and frail pulse.

■ **Cautions and Contraindications**

It is contraindicated in cases of excessive menses or uterine bleeding due to heat in the blood with bright red blood.

■ **Modern Applications**

Chronic functional uterine bleeding, threatened abortion, habitual abortion, postpartum bleeding, peptic ulcer, hemorrhoids, etc.

Jiao Tai Wan-Grand Communication Pill
Coptis and Cinnamon Formula
交泰丸

■ **Ingredients**

Huang Lian	Coptis	18g
Rou Gui	Cinnamon Bark	3g

■ **Preparation**

Use as prepared form or decoction.

■ **Pertaining Category**

Additional Formulas for Internal Medicine

■ **Functions**

Harmonizes the heart and kidney.

■ **Indications**

Disharmony between the heart and kidney manifested as irritability, restlessness, palpitation, coolness of lower limbs, severe insomnia, pale swollen tongue with thin white moist coat, a deep, weak pulse.

■ **Cautions and Contraindications**
None noted.

■ **Modern Applications**
Neurasthenia, heart disease, menopausal syndrome, etc.

Jie Yu Dan-Relieve Slurred Speech Elixir
Typhonium and Sweetflag Combination
解 语 丹

■ **Ingredients**

Bai Fu Zi	Typhonium	6g
Shi Chang Pu	Sweetflag Rhizome	6g
Yuan Zhi	Polygala Root	6g
Tian Ma	Gastrodia	9g
Quan Xie	Scorpion	3g
Qiang Huo	Notopterygium	6g
Tian Nan Xing	Arisaema Tuber	6g
Mu Xiang	Saussurea	6g
Gan Cao	Licorice	6g

■ **Preparation**
Use as prepared form or decoction.

■ **Pertaining Category**
Internal Wind Extinguishing

■ **Functions**
Extinguishes wind, resolves phlegm, clears the orifices and collaterals, relieves slurred speech.

■ **Indications**
Aphasia due to wind-phlegm obstructing the orifices and collateral manifested as stiffness of the tongue and slurred speech, numbness of limbs, white moist tongue coat, a wiry, slippery pulse.

Cautions and Contraindications

■ **Cautions and Contraindications**

It is contraindicated during pregnancy.

■ **Modern Applications**

Sequelae of stroke, etc.

Jin Gui Shen Qi Wan-Tonify Kidney Qi Pill from Golden Cabinet
Rehmannia Eight Formula
金柜肾气丸

■ **Ingredients**

Shu Di Huang	Cooked Rehmannia	24g
Shan Zhu Yu	Dogwood Fruit	12g
Shan Yao	Dioscorea	12g
Ze Xie	Alisma	9g
Fu Ling	Hoelen/Poria	9g
Mu Dan Pi	Moutan Bark	9g
Fu Zi	Prepared Aconite	3g
Gui Zhi	Cinnamon Twig	3g

■ **Preparation**

Use as decoction or prepared form.

■ **Pertaining Category**

Yang Tonifying

■ **Functions**

Warms the kidney Yang, tonifies the kidney Qi.

■ **Indications**
Deficiency of the kidney Yang and Qi manifested as soreness and
weakness of lower back and lower limbs with cold sensation,
spasmodic pain in the lower abdomen, difficult or frequent
urination, or incontinence, impotence, seminal emission, phlegm-
fluid syndrome, diabetes, flaccidity of lower limbs, pale and swollen
tongue with white coat, a deep, weak pulse.

■ **Cautions and Contraindications**
It is contraindicated in cases of deficient fire due to Yin deficiency,
consumption of body fluid from dry heat.

■ **Modern Applications**
Chronic nephritis, diabetes, hypothyroidism, neurasthenia, chronic
bronchitis or asthma, pulmonary emphysema, menopausal syndrome
infertility, chronic consumptive diseases, etc.

Jin Ling Zi San-Melia Toosandan Powder
Melia and Corydalis Formula
金 铃 子 散

■ **Ingredients**

| Jin Ling Zi(Chuan Lian Zi) | Melia | 30g |
| Yan Hu Suo(Yuan Hu) | Corydalis | 30g |

■ **Preparation**
Use as prepared form or decoction with properly reduced dosage.

■ **Pertaining Category**
Qi Regulating (Moving)

■ **Functions**
Moves Qi, smoothes the liver. Clears heat. Promotes blood
circulation, stops pain.

Indications
Liver Qi stagnation turning to heat manifested as hypochondriac, epigastric, and abdominal pain, irritability, a bitter taste in the mouth, red tongue with yellow coat, a wiry, rapid pulse.

Cautions and Contraindications
Use with extreme caution during pregnancy.

Modern Applications
Chronic gastritis, hepatitis, cholecystitis, costal neuralgia, peptic ulcer, dysmenorrhea, etc.

Jin Suo Gu Jing Wan-Golden Lock Essence Stabilizing Pill
Lotus Stamen Formula
金 锁 固 精 丸

Ingredients

Sha Yuan Ji Li	Astragalus seed	60g
Qian Shi	Euryale Seed	60g
Long Gu	Dragon Bone	30g
Mu Li	Oyster Shell	30g
Lian Zi	Lotus Seed	60-120g
Lian Xu	Lotus Stamen	60g

Preparation
Use as prepared form or decoction with properly reduced dosage.

Pertaining Category
Binding the Essence to Stop Seminal Emission and Enuresis

Functions
Consolidates the kidneys, binds up essence.

■   Indications

Deficiency of the kidney Yang with inability of consolidating essence manifested as spermatorrhea, nocturnal emission, impotence soreness and weakness of lower back and knees, tinnitus, listlessness lassitude, frequent urination, poor appetite, pale tongue with white coat, a thin, weak pulse.

■   Cautions and Contraindications

It is contraindicated in cases of seminal emission due to damp-heat in the lower burner. It should be modified when used for seminal emission due to hyperactivity of fire from kidney Yin deficiency.

■   Modern Applications

Spermatorrhea, nocturnal emission, sexual dysfunction, neurasthenia etc.

This formula is primarily astringent, more kidney tonics should be used either with this formula or after seminal emission stopped.

Jing Fang Bai Du San-Schizonepeta and Sile Powder to Overcome Toxicity

Schizonepeta and Siler Formula

荆 防 败 毒 散

Ingredients

Jing Jie	Schizonepeta	4.5g
Fang Feng	Siler	4.5g
Qiang Huo	Notopterygium	4.5g
Du Huo	Tuhuo	4.5g
Chai Hu	Bupleurum	4.5g
Qian Hu	Hogfennel Root	4.5g
Zhi Ke	Bitter Orange	4.5g
Jie Geng	Platycodon	4.5g
Chuan Xiong	Ligusticum	4.5g
Sheng Jiang	Fresh ginger	3g
Bo He	Peppermint	4.5g
Gan Cao	Licorice	1.5g
Fu Ling	Hoelen/Poria	4.5g

Preparation

Use as decoction or prepared form. Bo He should be added 5
minutes near the end of cooking.

Pertaining Category

Pungent Warm Exterior Relieving

Functions

Promotes sweat, expels wind-cold-dampness, releases the exterior.
Reduces swelling, stops pain.

Indications

Invasion of wind-cold-dampness with strong constitution
manifested as aversion to cold, fever, absence of sweating,
headache, neck stiffness and pain, generalized body aches and
heaviness, or early stage of abscesses, carbuncles, furuncles, and
sores with redness, swelling, and pain, thin white tongue coat, a
superficial, rapid pulse.

■ Cautions and Contraindications
It should not be used for patients with weak constitution.

■ Modern Applications
Common cold, influenza, tonsillitis, parotitis, mastitis, acute dysentery, measles, or German measles, suppurative skin infection, hordeolum, etc.
This formula is modified from Ren Shen Bai Du San (Ginseng Overcome Toxicity Powder).

Jiu Wei Qiang Huo Tang-Nine Ingredients Qiang Huo Decoction
Notopterygium Combination
九 味 羌 活 汤

■ Ingredients

Qiang Huo	*Notopterygium*	5g
Fang Feng	*Siler*	5g
Cang Zhu	*Atractylodes*	5g
Xi Xin	*Asarum*	1g
Chuan Xiong	*Ligusticum*	3g
Bai Zhi	*Angelica Root*	3g
Sheng Di Huang	*Dried Rehmannia*	3g
Huang Qin	*Scute*	3g
Gan Cao	*Licorice*	3g

■ Preparation
Use as decoction or prepared form.

■ Pertaining Category
Pungent Warm Exterior Relieving

■ Functions
Promotes sweat, dispels wind-dampness, releases the exterior, alleviates pain. Clears interior heat.

■   Indications

Invasion of wind-cold-dampness with mild internal heat manifested
as aversion to wind-cold, fever, absence of sweating, headache,
neck stiffness, generalized body aches, slight thirst, a bitter taste in
the mouth, normal or red tongue with thin yellow coat, a superficial,
slippery, or rapid pulse.

■   Cautions and Contraindications

It is contraindicated in cases of patients with Qi and Yin deficiency.
Do not use overdose and for long term.

■   Modern Applications

Common cold, influenza, rheumatic arthritis, acute lower back pain,
sinusitis, etc.
This formula is from "Ci Shi Nan Zhi "(Hard-won Knowledge).

Jiu Xian San-Nine Immortal Powder
九仙散

■   Ingredients

Ren Shen	Ginseng	2g
Kuan Dong Hua	Coltsfoot Flower	2g
Jie Geng	Platycodon	2g
Sang Bai Pi	Mulberry Rootbark	2g
Wu Wei Zi	Schisandra	2g
E Jiao	Equus/Gelatin	2g
Chuan Bei Mu	Tendrilled Fritillary	2g
Wu Mei	Black Plum	6g
Ying Su Ke	Papaver	6g
Sheng Jiang	Fresh Ginger	1slice
Da Zao	Jujube	1pc

■   Preparation

Use as decoction or prepared form. E Jiao should be dissolved
separately in boiling water and added into the strained decoction.

■ **Pertaining Category**
Stabilizing the Lungs to Stop Coughing

■ **Functions**
Tonifies the lung Qi, nourishes the lung Yin. Astringes the lungs, stops coughing.

■ **Indications**
Lung Qi and Yin deficiency manifested as prolonged cough, shortness of breath with wheezing, spontaneous sweating, general fatigue, pale tongue with thin white coat, a thin, weak, or rapid pulse.

■ **Cautions and Contraindications**
It is contraindicated in cases of cough associated with exterior patterns or excessive phlegm-damp retention.

■ **Modern Applications**
Chronic consumptive diseases, pulmonary tuberculosis, chronic bronchitis, etc.

Ju He Wan-Tangerine Seed Pill
Tangerine Seed Formula
橘 核 丸

■ Ingredients

Ju He	Tangerine Seed	30g
Chuan Lian Zi	Melia	30g
Tao Ren	Peach Kernel	30g
Hou Po	Magnolia Bark	15g
Mu Tong	Akebia	15g
Zhi Shi	Immature Citrus	15g
Yan Hu Suo	Corydalis	15g
Rou Gui	Cinnamon Bark	15g
Mu Xiang	Saussurea	15g
Hai Zao	Sargassum	30g
Kun Bu	Kelp Thallus	30g
Hai Dai	Laminaria	30g

■ Preparation
Use as prepared form or decoction with properly reduced dosage.

■ Pertaining Category
Qi Regulating(Moving)

■ Functions
Moves Qi, stops pain. Softens hardening, disperses lumps.

■ Indications
Stagnation of Qi, blood, and phlegm-damp in the liver channel and lower burner due to damp-cold manifested as hernial pain in the lower abdomen, swollen testis with a bearing down sensation, hard mass and nodules, swelling of the scrotum, pale tongue with white greasy coat, a deep, wiry, and slow pulse.

■ Cautions and Contraindications
Do not use this formula with overdose and for long term.

■ Modern Applications
Hernia, orchitis, epididymitis, hydrocele, etc.

Ju Pi Zhu Ru Tang-Tangerine Peel and Bamboo Shaving Decoction
Aurantium and Bamboo Combination
橘皮竹茹汤

■ **Ingredients**

Ju Pi	Tangerine Peel	9-12g
Zhu Ru	Bamboo Shaving	9-12g
Ren Shen	Ginseng	3g
Sheng Jiang	Fresh Ginger	6-9g
Da Zao	Jujube	5pcs
Gan Cao	Licorice	3-6g

■ **Preparation**

Use as decoction or prepared form.

■ **Pertaining Category**

Qi Regulating(Descending)

■ **Functions**

Descends the rebellious stomach Qi, stops vomiting. Tonifies Qi. Clears heat.

■ **Indications**

Heat in the stomach with deficient and rebellious stomach Qi manifested as nausea, vomiting, or hiccups, retch, poor appetite, or dry mouth, light red tongue, a thin, weak, rapid pulse.

■ **Cautions and Contraindications**

It is contraindicated in cases of vomiting and hiccups due to excess heat or deficient cold.

■ **Modern Applications**

Gastritic vomiting, neurogenic vomiting, morning sickness, pyloristenosis, pylorospasm, hiccups after abdominal operation, etc.

Ju Yuan Jian-Lift the Source Brew
Ginseng and Cimicifuga Formula
举 元 煎

■ **Ingredients**

Ren Shen	Ginseng	9g
Huang Qi	Astragalus	9-15g
Bai Zhu	White Atractylodes	6-9g
Zhi Gan Cao	Baked Licorice	3-6g
Sheng Ma	Cimicifuga	4g

■ **Preparation**
Use as decoction or prepared form.

■ **Pertaining Category**
Qi Tonifying

■ **Functions**
Tonifies and lifts the Qi, stabilizes menses, stops uterine bleeding.

■ **Indications**
Spleen Qi deficiency and sinking manifested as severe uterine bleeding which is pale in color and thin quality, shortness of breath, palpitation, pale complexion, fatigue, a sinking sensation in the lower abdomen, or cold limbs and cold sweats, pale and swollen tongue with thin white moist coat, a weak, frail pulse.

■ **Cautions and Contraindications**
It is contraindicated in cases of uterine bleeding due to excess heat.

■ **Modern Applications**
Uterine bleeding, gastroptosis, prolapse of the rectum and uterus, etc.

Juan Bi Tang-Alleviating Painful Obstruction Decoction

Chianghuo and Turmeric Combination

蠲痹汤

■ **Ingredients**

Qiang Huo	Notopterygium	9g
Jiang Huang	Turmeric Rhizome	9g
Dang Gui	Chinese Angelica	9g
Chi Shao Yao	Red Peony	9g
Fang Feng	Siler	9g
Huang Qi	Astragalus	9g
Zhi Gan Cao	Baked Licorice	3g
Sheng Jiang	Fresh Ginger	3g

■ **Preparation**
Use as decoction or prepared form.

■ **Pertaining Category**
Wind-dampness Expelling

■ **Functions**
Expels wind-dampness, alleviates pain. Tonifies Qi, harmonizes blood.

■ **Indications**
Painful bi syndrome due to wind-dampness invasion with Qi deficiency manifested as pain and heaviness of body mostly in the neck, shoulder, and upper limbs with numbness sensation, slight joint swelling, pale tongue with thin white coat, a superficial, slight slow, and soft pulse.

■ **Cautions and Contraindications**
None noted.

■ **Modern Applications**
Rheumatic arthritis, osteoarthritis, frozen shoulder, etc.
This formula is from "Bai Yi Xuan Fang" (Selected Formulas).

Kai Yu Zhong Yu Tang-Open Depression and Plant Jade Decoction

开郁种玉汤

■ **Ingredients**

Dang Gui	Chinese Angelica	12g
Bai Shao Yao	White Peony	12g
Bai Zhu	White Atractylodes	9g
Fu Ling	Hoelen/Poria	9g
Mu Dan Pi	Moutan Bark	9g
Xiang Fu	Cyperus Tuber	9g
Tian Hua Fen	Trichosanthes	9g

■ **Preparation**

Use as decoction or prepared form.

■ **Pertaining Category**

Additional Formulas for Ob-Gyn Disorders

■ **Functions**

Soothes the liver, moves Qi, relieves depression. Nourishes blood, normalizes menses. Strengthens the spleen.

■ **Indications**

Infertility due to liver Qi stagnation manifested as inability to conceive, irregular menstruation, difficult, scanty, dark colored menses with blood clots and menstrual cramps, premenstrual breast distention and abdominal bloating, irritability, or mental depression, dark red or purple tongue with thin white coat, a wiry pulse.

■ **Cautions and Contraindications**

None noted.

■ **Modern Applications**

Infertility, irregular menstruation, dysmenorrhea, premenstrual syndrome, etc.

Ke Xue Fang-Coughing of Blood Formula
Indigo and Trichosanthes Formula
咳血方

■ **Ingredients**

Qing Dai	Indigo	6-9g
Gua Lou Ren	Trichosanthes	9g
Hai Fu Shi	Pumice	9g
Zhi Zi	Gardenia Fruit	9g
He Zi	Myrobalan Fruit	6-9g

■ **Preparation**
Use as decoction or prepared form.

■ **Pertaining Category**
Stopping Bleeding

■ **Functions**
Clears the liver fire, resolves phlegm. Preserves the lungs, stops coughing and bleeding.

■ **Indications**
Liver fire attacking the lungs manifested as cough with blood-tinged thick sputum that is difficult to expectorate, irritability, easily to get angry, stabbing pain in the chest and hypochondrium, red complexion, a bitter taste in the mouth, thirst, constipation, red tongue with yellow coat, a wiry, rapid pulse.

■ **Cautions and Contraindications**
Use with caution for patients with deficiency of the spleen and stomach.

■ **Modern Applications**
Bronchiectasis, pulmonary tuberculosis, etc.

Kong Yan Dan-Control Mucus Elixir
Kansui and Brassica Formula
控涎丹

■   **Ingredients**

Gan Sui Da Ji Bai Jie Zi	*Kansui Root* *Euphorbia* *Brassica Seed*	Equal dosage

■   **Preparation**
Grind all ingredients into fine powder and make small pills, take 1-3g each time.

■   **Pertaining Category**
Purging Downward with Harsh Cathartics

■   **Functions**
Resolves phlegm, eliminates water retention.

■   **Indications**
Phlegm retaining above and below the diaphragm and obstructing the Qi manifested as sudden, unbearable pain in the neck, thorax, and lower back, tightening and burning pain in the joints, or cold limbs, or severe headache, or lethargy, tastelessness, coughing with thick, sticky sputum, a rattling sound in the throat during night, profuse salivation, greasy tongue coat, a wiry, slippery pulse.

■   **Cautions and Contraindications**
It is contraindicated for patients with weak constitution or during pregnancy. If severe diarrhea occurs, the cold rice porridge should be taken to benefit recovery.

■   **Modern Applications**
Pleural effusion, uremia from systemic lupus erythematosus, nephritic syndrome, ascites from cirrhosis or late stage of schistosomiasis, etc.

Li Zhong An Hui Tang-Regulate the Middle Burner and Calm Roundworms Decoction

Atractylodes and Black Plum Combination

理中安蛔汤

■ Ingredients

Ren Shen	Ginseng	2.1g
Bai Zhu	White Atractylodes	3g
Fu Ling	Hoelen/Poria	3g
Hua Jiao	Zanthoxylum	0.9g
Wu Mei	Black Plum	0.9g
Gan Jiang	Dried Ginger	1.5g

■ Preparation
Use as decoction or prepared form.

■ Pertaining Category
Parasites Expelling

■ Functions
Warms the middle burner, tonifies the spleen Qi, calms roundworms.

■ Indications
Deficient cold in the spleen and stomach with roundworm disturbance manifested as loose stools or diarrhea, abdominal pain, borborygmus, profuse and clear urine, cold limbs, vomiting of roundworms or passing roundworms in the watery stools, pale tongue with thin white coat, a slow, weak pulse.

■ Cautions and Contraindications
It is contraindicated in cases of roundworms with heat signs.

■ Modern Applications
Ascariasis, biliary ascariasis, chronic gastroenteritis, etc.

Li Zhong Wan-Regulate the Middle Burner Pill

Ginseng and Ginger Combination
理 中 丸

■ Ingredients

Ren Shen	Ginseng	6g
Gan Jiang	Dried Ginger	5g
Bai Zhu	White Atractylodes	9g
Zhi Gan Cao	Baked Licorice	6g

■ Preparation
Use as prepared form or decoction.

■ Pertaining Category
Middle Burner Warming and Cold Dispelling

■ Functions
Warms the middle burner, dispels cold. Tonifies spleen and stomach Qi.

■ Indications
Qi and Yang deficiency of the spleen and stomach with internal cold manifested as abdominal pain which is alleviated by warmth and hand pressure, watery diarrhea, abdominal distention, clear urine, absence of thirst, lack of appetite, vomiting clear fluid or spitting saliva, fullness in the chest, or chronic infantile convulsion, pale tongue with white coat, a deep, thin pulse.

■ Cautions and Contraindications
It is contraindicated in cases of exterior wind-heat invasion or interior heat with Yin deficiency.

■ Modern Applications
Chronic gastritis and enteritis, peptic ulcer, chronic colitis, indigestion, gastric dilatation, gastroptosis, cholera, etc.

Liang Fu Wan-Galanga and Cyperus Pill
Galanga and Cyperus Formula
良 附 丸

■ **Ingredients**

| Gao Liang Jiang | *Galanga* | 6-9g |
| Xiang Fu | *Cyperus* | 6-9g |

■ **Preparation**

Use as prepared form or decoction.

■ **Pertaining Category**

Qi Regulating(Moving)

■ **Functions**

Promotes the free flowing of liver Qi. Warms the middle burner, dispels cold, stops pain.

■ **Indications**

Liver Qi stagnation with cold in the stomach manifested as epigastric and abdominal pain that is alleviated by warmth, vomiting, fullness and distending pain in the chest and hypochondrium, pale tongue with white coat, a wiry, slow pulse.

■ **Cautions and Contraindications**

It is contraindicated in cases of stomachalgia or vomiting due to heat.

■ **Modern Applications**

Chronic gastritis, peptic ulcer, etc.

Liang Ge San-Cool the Diaphragm Powder
Forsythia and Rhubarb Formula
凉 膈 散

- **Ingredients**

Da Huang	Rhubarb	600g
Mang Xiao	Mirabilitum	600g
Zhi Zi	Gardenia Fruit	300g
Huang Qin	Scute	300g
Bo He	Peppermint	300g
Lian Qiao	Forsythia Fruit	1200g
Gan Cao	Licorice	600g
Dan Zhu Ye	Bland Bamboo Leaf	Proper amount

- **Preparation**

Use as prepared form or decoction with properly reduced dosage.

- **Pertaining Category**

Heat Clearing and Detoxicating

- **Functions**

Purges fire-heat from upper and middle burners, promotes bowel movement, relieves toxicity.

- **Indications**

Excessive fire-heat accumulating in the upper and middle burners manifested as fever, irritable heat in the chest and diaphragm region, or even delirium, thirst, red face, dry and chapped lips, ulceration of the mouth and tongue, sore throat, or vomiting of blood, nosebleeding, constipation or hesitant bowel movement, scanty and dark urine, red tongue with yellow coat, a slippery, rapid pulse.

- **Cautions and Contraindications**

It is contraindicated in cases of the spleen and stomach Yang deficiency or Yin deficiency with deep-red and uncoated tongue.

- **Modern Applications**

Influenza, encephalitis B, meningitis, septicemia, pyogenic skin infection, hepatitis, acute gastroenteritis or dysentery, acute UTI, acute cholecystitis, as well as stomatitis, toothache, and laryngopharyngitis, etc.

This formula is modified from Tiao Wei Cheng Qi Tang (Regulate Stomach Decoction for Purging Downward Digestive Qi).

Ling Gan Wu Wei Jiang Xin Tang-Poria, Licorice, Schisandra, Ginger, and Asarum Decoction
Hoelen and Schisandra Combination
苓甘五味姜辛汤

■ **Ingredients**

Fu Ling	Hoelen/Poria	12g
Gan Jiang	Dried Ginger	9g
Xi Xin	Asarum	3g
Wu Wei Zi	Schisandra	6g
Gan Cao	Licorice	6g

■ **Preparation**
Use as decoction or prepared form.

■ **Pertaining Category**
Cold-phlegm Transforming

■ **Functions**
Warms the lungs, transforms phlegm-fluid.

■ **Indications**
Cold-phlegm fluid retaining in the lungs with spleen Yang deficiency manifested as cough and wheezing with profuse white clear sputum, fullness and discomfort in the chest and diaphragm, or salivation, pale tongue with white moist tongue coat, a wiry, slippery, or weak pulse.

■ Cautions and Contraindications

It is contraindicated in cases of cough or asthma due to lung heat, phlegm-fire, dryness in the lungs, and lung Yin deficiency. Do not use overdose and for long term.

■ Modern Applications

Chronic bronchitis, bronchial asthma, pulmonary emphysema, chronic obstructive pulmonary disease, etc.

Ling Gui Zhu Gan Tang-Poria, Cinnamon, Atractylodes, and Licorice Decoction
Hoelen and Atractylodes Combination
苓 桂 术 甘 汤

■ Ingredients

Fu Ling	Hoelen/Poria	12g
Gui Zhi	Cinnamon Twig	9g
Bai Zhu	White Atractylodes	6g
Zhi Gan Cao	Baked Licorice	6g

■ Preparation

Use as decoction or prepared form.

■ Pertaining Category

Yang Warming and Dampness Transforming

■ Functions

Warms Yang, transforms phlegm-fluid. Tonifies the spleen Qi, drains dampness.

■ **Indications**

Phlegm-fluid retention affecting the upper or middle burner with spleen Yang deficiency manifested as cough with clear watery sputum, difficulty in breathing, shortness of breath, a fullness sensation in the chest and hypochondrium, dizziness, vertigo, palpitation, or nausea, pale tongue with white moist coat, a wiry, slippery, or deep, weak pulse.

■ **Cautions and Contraindications**

It is contraindicated in cases of Yin deficiency.

■ **Modern Applications**

Chronic bronchitis, bronchial asthma, pulmonary emphysema, Meniere's syndrome, vegetative (Autonomic) nerve dysfunction, tinnitus, cardiac or nephritis edema, chronic gastritis, chronic nephritis, etc.

Ling Jiao Gou Teng Tang-Antelope Horn and Uncaria Decoction
Antelope Horn and Uncaria Combination
羚 角 钩 藤 汤

■ **Ingredients**

Ling Yang Jiao	Antelope Horn	4.5g
Sang Ye	Mulberry Leaf	6g
Chuan Bei Mu	Tendrilled Fritillary	12g
Sheng Di Huang	Dried Rehmannia	15g
Gou Teng	Uncaria	9g
Ju Hua	Chrysanthemum	9g
Bai Shao Yao	White Peony	9g
Zhu Ru	Bamboo Shavings	15g
Fu Shen	Hoelen/Poria	9g
Gan Cao	Licorice	2.4g

■ **Preparation**

Use as decoction. Ling Yang Jiao should be decocted first for one hour prior to other herbs; Gou Teng should be added near the end; or add Ling Yang Jiao as a powder to the strained decoction. Ling Yang Jiao can be substituted by Zhen Zhu Mu (Mother of Pearl Shell). This formula is also available as prepared form.

■ **Pertaining Category**

Internal Wind Extinguishing

■ **Functions**

Clears the liver heat, subdues the liver Yang, extinguishes wind. Generates body fluid to relax muscles and tendons.

■ **Indications**

Extreme liver heat stirring up wind manifested as persistent high fever, irritability, restlessness, or delirium and convulsion, or even coma, dark red and dry tongue with prickles, a wiry, rapid pulse.

■ **Cautions and Contraindications**

It is contraindicated in cases of tremors and convulsion due to Yin or blood deficiency.

■ **Modern Applications**

Hypertension, cerebrovascular accident, epilepsy, hyperthyroidism, vertigo, encephalitis B, epidemic cerebral-spinal meningitis, etc.

Liu Jun Zi Tang-Six Gentleman Decoction
Six Major Herb Combination
六 君 子 汤

■ Ingredients

Ren Shen	Ginseng	9g
Bai Zhu	White Atractylodes	9g
Fu Ling	Hoelen/Poria	9g
Chen Pi	Tangerine Peel	9g
Ban Xia	Pinellia Tuber	12g
Zhi Gan Cao	Baked Licorice	6g

■ Preparation
Use as decoction or prepared form.

■ Pertaining Category
Qi Tonifying

■ Functions
Tonifies the spleen Qi, transforms dampness, resolves phlegm, stops vomiting.

■ Indications
Spleen and stomach Qi deficiency with phlegm-dampness retention manifested as poor appetite, nausea, vomiting, fullness in the chest and epigastrium, loose stools, or cough with profuse, white, thin sputum, pale tongue with white coat, a soft, weak pulse.

■ Cautions and Contraindications
It is contraindicated in cases of high fever, empty fire, bloating due to food stagnation, lack of body fluid, excessive thirst, constipation. Long term use may cause thirst, dryness of tongue or mouth, and irritability.

■ Modern Applications
Chronic gastroenteritis, peptic ulcer, sour regurgitation, indigestion, chronic bronchitis, morning sickness, etc.

Liu Mo Tang-Six Milled Herbs Decoction
Aquilaria and Rhubarb Combination
六 磨 汤

■ **Ingredients**

Chen Xiang	Aquilaria	3g
Mu Xiang	Saussurea	6g
Bing Lang	Betel Nut	9g
Wu Yao	Lindera Root	6g
Da Huang	Rhubarb	9g
Zhi Shi	Immature Citrus	6g

■ **Preparation**
Use as decoction or prepared form. Da Huang should be added 5 minutes near the end of making decoction.

■ **Pertaining Category**
Additional Formulas for Internal Medicine

■ **Functions**
Moves Qi, promotes bowel movement.

■ **Indications**
Qi stagnation leading to constipation accompanied with frequent belching, a fullness sensation in the chest and hypochondrium, abdominal distention or pain, reduced appetite, thin greasy tongue coat, a wiry pulse.

■ **Cautions and Contraindications**
It is contraindicated during pregnancy and in cases of constipation due to deficiency.

■ **Modern Applications**
Constipation, etc.

Liu Wei Di Huang Wan-Six Ingredients Pill with Rehmannia

Rehmannia Six Formula
六味地黄丸

■ **Ingredients**

Shu Di Huang	*Cooked Rehmannia*	24g
Shan Zhu Yu	*Dogwood Fruit*	12g
Shan Yao	*Dioscorea*	12g
Fu Ling	*Hoelen/Poria*	9g
Ze Xie	*Alisma*	9g
Mu Dan Pi	*Moutan Bark*	9g

■ **Preparation**
Use as prepared form or decoction.

■ **Pertaining Category**
Yin Tonifying

■ **Functions**
Nourishes the liver and kidney Yin.

■ **Indications**
Yin deficiency of the liver and kidney manifested as soreness and weakness of lower back and knees, dizziness, blurred vision, tinnitus, deafness, night sweats, nocturnal emission, tidal or steaming bone fever, a feverish sensation in the palms and soles, or toothache, dry mouth and throat, or delayed closing of fontanel in children, red tongue with scanty coat, a thin, rapid pulse.

■ **Cautions and Contraindications**

Use with extreme caution for patients with indigestion and diarrhea due to deficiency of the spleen and stomach.

■ **Modern Applications**

Diabetes, hypertension, arteriosclerosis, hyperthyroidism, neurasthenia, chronic nephritis, chronic pyelonephritis, pulmonary tuberculosis, optic neuritis or atrophy, infantile dysplasia, amenorrhea, menopausal syndrome, etc.

Liu Yi San-Six to One Powder
Talcum and Licorice
六 一 散

■ **Ingredients**

Hua Shi	Talcum	180g
Gan Cao	Licorice	30g

■ **Preparation**

Use as prepared form or decoction with properly reduced dosage.

■ **Pertaining Category**

Summer Heat Clearing

■ **Functions**

Clears summer heat, drains dampness.

■ **Indications**

Summer heat with dampness manifested as fever, irritability, thirst, difficult urination, or diarrhea, or vomiting, thin yellow greasy tongue coat, a slippery, rapid pulse.

■ Cautions and Contraindications
Use with caution for elderly or patients with Qi and Yin deficiency.

■ Modern Applications
Summer diarrhea, acute UTI, etc.

Long Dan Xie Gan Tang-Gentiana Drain the Liver Decoction
Gentiana Combination
龙 胆 泻 肝 汤

■ Ingredients

Long Dan Cao	Gentiana	6g
Huang Qin	Scute	9g
Zhi Zi	Gardenia Fruit	9g
Ze Xie	Alisma	12g
Mu Tong	Akebia	9g
Che Qian Zi	Plantago Seed	9g
Dang Gui	Chinese Angelica	3g
Sheng Di Huang	Dried Rehmannia	9g
Chai Hu	Bupleurum	6g
Gan Cao	Licorice	6g

■ Preparation
Use as decoction or prepared form. Che Qian Zi should be wrapped in gauze when making decoction.

■ Pertaining Category
Clearing Heat from Zang-fu Organs

■ Functions
Purges excessive fire and dam-heat from liver and gallbladder. Eliminates damp-heat from lower burner.

■ Indications

Liver fire flaring up or liver and gallbladder damp-heat flowing down to lower burner manifested as headache, red, swelling, and painful eyes, irritability, easy to get angry, a bitter taste in the mouth, dry throat, hypochondriac pain, ear swollen and pain, or deaf, itching, swelling, or sweating around the external genitals, scanty and difficult urination, thick, yellow, and foul smelling vaginal discharge, red tongue with yellow greasy coat, a wiry, slippery, and rapid pulse.

■ Cautions and Contraindications

Use with extreme caution for patients with deficiency of the spleen and stomach. Avoid overdose and long-term administration.

■ Modern Applications

Acute conjunctivitis, acute ear infection, acute cholecystitis, herpes zoster, acute cystitis, acute UTI, acute pelvic inflammation, acute prostatitis, scrotal eczema, cholelithiasis, orchitis, erysipelas, hyperthyroidism, etc.

Ma Huang Fu Zi Xi Xin Tang-Ephedra, Aconite, and Asarum Decoction
Ma Huang and Asarum Combination
麻黄附子细辛汤

■ Ingredients

Ma Huang	Ephedra	6g
Fu Zi	Prepared Aconite	9g
Xi Xin	Asarum	3g

■ Preparation

Use as decoction or prepared form.

■ Pertaining Category

Strengthening Body Resistance and Relieving Exterior

■ Functions
Warms Yang Qi, expels wind-cold, releases the exterior.

■ Indications
Invasion of wind-cold with Yang deficiency manifested as severe aversion to cold, slight fever without sweating, the chills relieved by wearing more clothing or adding covers, pale and moist tongue with white coat, a deep, weak pulse.

■ Cautions and Contraindications
Only use this formula for patient with exterior wind-cold with underlying Yang deficiency.

■ Modern Applications
Common cold, edema from nephritis, chronic pulmonary heart disease, etc.

Ma Huang Tang-Ephedra Decoction
Ma Huang Combination
麻黄汤

■ Ingredients

Ma Huang	Ephedra	9g
Gui Zhi	Cinnamon Twig	6g
Xing Ren	Apricot Seed	9g
Zhi Gan Cao	Baked Licorice	3g

■ Preparation
Use as decoction or prepared form.

■ Pertaining Category
Pungent Warm Exterior Relieving

■ Functions
Promotes sweat, dispels wind-cold, releases the exterior. Facilitates the lung Qi, relieves asthma.

■ Indications

Exterior wind-cold invasion manifested as severe aversion to cold, mild fever, headache, body aches, absence of sweating, wheezing, thin white tongue coat, a superficial, tight pulse.

■ Cautions and Contraindications

It is contraindicated in cases of exterior deficiency with spontaneous sweating, exterior wind-heat, and weak constitution. Use with caution for patients with hypertension and heart problems.

■ Modern Applications

Common cold, influenza, upper respiratory tract infection, bronchitis, bronchial asthma, and acute glomerulonephritis, etc. *This formula has strong effect of inducing sweats. It should be withdrawn immediately as soon as patient perspired and the illness is cured.*

Ma Huang Xing Ren Gan Cao Shi Gao Tang-Ephedra, Apricot Seed, Licorice, and Gypsum Decoction
Ma Huang And Apricot Seed Combination
麻黄杏仁甘草石膏汤

■ Ingredients

Ma Huang	*Ephedra*	5g
Xing Ren	*Apricot Seed*	9g
Shi Gao	*Gypsum*	18g
Zhi Gan Cao	*Baked Licorice*	6g

■ Preparation

Use as decoction or prepared form.

- **Pertaining Category**

Pungent Cool Exterior Relieving

- **Functions**

Disperses lung Qi, clears lung heat, directs rebellious Qi downward, stops coughing and wheezing.

- **Indications**

Excessive heat in the lungs manifested as persistent fever with or without sweating, or slight chills, cough with dyspnea or even accompanied by nasal flaring and chest pain, thirst, thin white or yellow tongue coat, slippery, rapid pulse.

- **Cautions and Contraindications**

It is contraindicated in cases of asthma due to cold or deficiency. Use with caution for patients with hypertension or heart problems.

- **Modern Applications**

Pneumonia, bronchitis, bronchial asthma, measles, whooping cough, upper respiratory tract infection, etc.

Ma Zi Ren Wan-Hemp Seed Pill
Apricot Seed and linum Formula
麻子仁丸

- **Ingredients**

Huo Ma Ren	Hemp Seed	500g
Bai Shao Yao	White Peony	250g
Zhi Shi	Immature Citrus	250g
Da Huang	Rhubarb	500g
Hou Po	Magnolia Bark	250g
Xing Ren	Apricot Seed	250g

- **Preparation**

Use as prepared form or decoction with properly reduced dosage.

- ■ **Pertaining Category**
Purging Downward with Moist Laxatives

- ■ **Functions**
Moistens the intestines, promotes bowel movement. Moves Qi circulation. Eliminates heat.

- ■ **Indications**
Pathogenic dry heat in the Yangming with lack of body fluid manifested as dry stool, frequent urination, or habitual constipation, red tongue with dry yellow coat, a thin, rapid or empty pulse.

- ■ **Cautions and Contraindications**
Do not use during pregnancy. Use with caution for elderly, weak constitution patients, as well as constipation due to deficiency of blood and Yin.

- ■ **Modern Applications**
Habitual constipation, hemorrhoids, postpartum or post-surgical constipation, anal fissure, etc.

Mai Men Dong Tang-Ophiopogon Decoction
Ophiopogon Formula
麦门冬汤

- ■ **Ingredients**

Mai Men Dong	Ophiopogon	6-12g
Ban Xia	Pinellia Tuber	6-9g
Ren Shen	Ginseng	6-9g
Geng Mi	Oryza	9-12g
Da Zao	Jujube	10pcs
Gan Cao	Licorice	3-6g

- ■ **Preparation**
Use as decoction or prepared form.

■ Pertaining Category
Moistening Dryness

■ Functions
Nourishes the lung and stomach Yin, moistens dryness. Descends the adverse flow of Qi. Tonifies Qi, harmonizes middle burner.

■ Indications
Lung and stomach Yin deficiency with rebellious and deficient Qi manifested as cough with sputum which is difficult to expectorate, or spitting of whitish frothy saliva, shortness of breath, nausea, vomiting, dry mouth and throat, thirst, a feverish sensation in the palms and soles, red tongue with scanty coat, a weak, thin, and rapid pulse.

■ Cautions and Contraindications
It is contraindicated for patients with consumptive lung disease due to deficient cold.

■ Modern Applications
Chronic bronchitis, bronchiectasis, pulmonary tuberculosis, chronic pharyngitis, chronic gastritis, atrophic gastritis, etc.

Mu Li San-Oyster Shell Powder
牡蛎散

■ Ingredients

Mu Li	Oyster Shell	15-30g
Huang Qi	Astragalus	9-15g
Ma Huang Gen	Ephedra Root	6-9g
Fu Xiao Mai	Light Wheat	15-30g

■ Preparation
Use as decoction or prepared form.

■ Pertaining Category
Consolidating Exterior to Stop Sweating

■ Functions
Consolidates defensive Qi, astringes the exterior to stop sweating. Nourishes heart.

■ Indications
Qi deficiency causing spontaneous and excessive sweating with further injury of heart Yin manifested as spontaneous sweating, worse at night, or night sweats, fatigue, listlessness, palpitation, irritable heat in the chest, dream disturbed sleep, easily frightened, shortness of breath, general debility, pale red tongue, a thin, weak pulse.

■ Cautions and Contraindications
It is inappropriate to use this formula for profuse or oily sweating due to collapse of Yang or Yin.

■ Modern Applications
Hyperhidrosis, night or spontaneous sweats, vegetative nerve dysfunction, chronic consumptive disease, etc.

Mu Xiang Bing Lang Wan-Aucklandia and Betel Nut Pill
Pills of Saussurea and Areca Seed
木香槟榔丸

- **Ingredients**

Mu Xiang	Saussurea	30g
Bing Lang	Betel Nut	30g
Qing Pi	Green Citurs Peel	30g
Chen Pi	Tangerine Peel	30g
Huang Lian	Coptis	30g
Huang Bai	Phellodendron Bark	30g
Xiang Fu	Cyperus Tuber	60g
Da Huang	Rhubarb	15g
E Zhu	Zedoaria	30g
Qian Niu Zi	Pharbitis Seed	60g

- **Preparation**

Use as prepared form or decoction with properly reduced dosage.

- **Pertaining Category**

Food Stagnation Relieving

- **Functions**

Moves Qi, improves digestion, removes stagnant food. Purges heat, promotes bowel movement.

- **Indications**

Severe food and Qi stagnation with damp-heat retention manifested as severe epigastric and abdominal distention and pain, dysentery with tenesmus, blood and mucus in the stools, or constipation, red tongue with yellow greasy coat, a deep, slippery, rapid, and forceful pulse.

- **Cautions and Contraindications**

It is contraindicated during pregnancy and for patients with weak constitution.

- **Modern Applications**

Acute gastroenteritis, acute dysentery, indigestion, acute or chronic cholecystitis, acute pancreatitis, hepatitis, etc.

231

Nei Bu Wan-Internal Tonification Pill
内补丸

■ **Ingredients**

Lu Rong	Pilose Deerhorn	1.5g
Tu Si Zi	Dodder Seed	12g
Sha Yuan Ji Li	Astragalus Seed	12g
Huang Qi	Astragalus Root	12g
Rou Gui	Cinnamon Bark	6g
Sang Piao Xiao	Mantis Egg-case	9g
Rou Cong Rong	Cistanche	12g
Zhi Fu Zi	Prepared Aconite	6g
Zi Wan	Purple Aster Root	9g
Ci Ji Li	Tribulus	9g

■ **Preparation**
Use as decoction or prepared form.

■ **Pertaining Category**
Yang Tonifying

■ **Functions**
Warms the kidney Yang, stops vaginal discharge.

■ **Indications**
Leukorrhea due to kidney Qi and Yang deficiency manifested as excessive, watery, and clear vaginal discharge, severs lower back pain, a cold sensation in the lower abdomen, frequent and clear urine, especially during night, loose stools, pale tongue with thin white coat, a deep, slower, and weak pulse.

■ **Cautions and Contraindications**
It is contraindicated in cases of excess or deficient heat patterns.

■ **Modern Applications**
Leukorrhea, infertility, lower back pain, etc.

Niu Bang Jie Ji Tang-Burdock Seed Release Muscle Decoction

Ligustrum Decoction to Expel Pathogen from Muscle
牛蒡解肌汤

■ Ingredients

Niu Bang Zi	*Burdock Seed*	10g
Bo He	*Peppermint*	6g
Jing Jie	*Schizonepeta*	6g
Lian Qiao	*Forsythia Fruit*	10g
Zhi Zi	*Gardenia Fruit*	10g
Mu Dan Pi	*Moutan Bark*	10g
Shi Hu	*Dendrobium*	12g
Xuan Shen	*Scrophularia Root*	10g
Xia Ku Cao	*Prunella Spike*	12g

■ Preparation
Use as decoction or prepared form.

■ Pertaining Category
Treating External Carbuncles

■ Functions
Expels wind, clears heat, cools blood, reduces swelling.

■ Indications
Localized carbuncles and boils due to toxic phlegm-heat accompanied with exterior wind-heat manifested as quickly developed redness, swelling, and pain in the head, face, and neck, toothache, severe sore throat, fever, mild chills, lack of sweating, thirst, yellow and scanty urine, thin white or yellow tongue coat, a superficial, rapid pulse.

■ Cautions and Contraindications
Use with caution for patients with spleen and stomach deficiency.

■ Modern Applications
Carbuncles, boils, scrofula, toothache, parotitis, acute tonsillitis, etc.

Niu Huang Qing Xin Wan-Clear the Heart Pill with Ox Gallstone

Ox Gallstone and Coptis Formula

牛黄清心丸

■ **Ingredients**

Niu Huang	Ox Gallstone	0.75g
Huang Lian	Coptis	15g
Huang Qin	Scute	9g
Zhi Zi	Gardenia Fruit	9g
Yu Jin	Curcuma Root	6g
Zhu Sha	Cinnabar	4.5g

■ **Preparation**
Use as prepared form.

■ **Pertaining Category**
Aromatically Opening Orifices with Cold Nature

■ **Functions**
Clears heat, relieves toxicity. Calms spirit. Opens orifices.

■ **Indications**
Heat penetrating the pericardium or phlegm-heat disturbing spirit manifested as fever, restlessness, delirium, impaired spirit, or coma, or infantile convulsion, red tongue with yellow greasy coat, a wiry, slippery, and rapid pulse.

■ **Cautions and Contraindications**
Do not use overdose and for long term. It is contraindicated during pregnancy.

■ **Modern Applications**
Encephalitis B, epidemic cerebral-spinal meningitis, cerebral vascular accident, urimia, toxic pneumonia, toxic dysentery, hepatic coma, infantile convulsions, etc.
This formula is weaker than An Gong Niu Huang Wan.

Nuan Gan Jian-Warm the Liver Brew
Lycium and Fennel Combination
暖肝煎

■ **Ingredients**

Dang Gui	Chinese Angelica	6-9g
Gou Qi Zi	Lycium fruit	9g
Xiao Hui Xiang	Fennel Fruit	6g
Rou Gui	Cinnamon Bark	3-6g
Wu Yao	Lindera	6g
Chen Xiang	Aquilaria	3g
Fu Ling	Hoelen/Poria	6g
Sheng Jiang	Fresh Ginger	3-5slices

■ **Preparation**
Use as decoction or prepared form.

■ **Pertaining Category**
Qi Regulating (Moving)

■ **Functions**
Warms the kidney Yang and liver channel, moves Qi, stops pain.

■ **Indications**
Kidney Qi and Yang deficiency with cold stagnation in the liver channel manifested as pain in the lower abdomen, hernia, swelling and pain of the scrotum, or impotence, or cramps prior to menses with a cold sensation in the lower abdomen, pale or purple tongue with white coat, a deep, wiry pulse.

■ **Cautions and Contraindications**
It is contraindicated in cases of pain, swelling, and redness of scrotum due to damp-heat in the lower burner.

■ **Modern Applications**
Inguinal hernia, hydrocele, epididymitis, varicocele, etc.

Ping Wei San-Calm the Stomach Powder
Magnolia and Ginger Formula
平胃散

■ **Ingredients**

Cang Zhu	Atractylodes	15g
Hou Po	Magnolia Bark	9g
Chen Pi	Tangerine Peel	9g
Gan Cao	Licorice	4g
Sheng Jiang	Fresh Ginger	2slices
Da Zao	Jujube	2pcs

■ **Preparation**
Use as decoction or prepared form.

■ **Pertaining Category**
Dampness Drying and Stomach Harmonizing

■ **Functions**
Dries dampness, strengthens the spleen. Moves Qi, harmonizes stomach.

■ **Indications**
Dampness obstructing Qi in the spleen and stomach manifested as fullness in the epigastrium, abdominal distention, poor appetite, tastelessness, or a sweet taste in the mouth, nausea, vomiting, belching, sour regurgitation, heaviness of body and limbs, lassitude, loose stools, white, thick, and greasy tongue coat, a slow, slippery pulse.

■ **Cautions and Contraindications**
It is contraindicated in cases of red tongue with scanty coat due to Yin deficiency or a bitter taste in the mouth, thirst, and rapid pulse due to excess heat.

■ **Modern Applications**
Acute and chronic gastroenteritis, catarrhal gastritis, gastrointestinal neurosis, indigestion, hepatitis, etc.

236

Pu Ji Xiao Du Yin-Universal Benefit Beverage to Relieve Toxicity
Scute and Cimicifuga Combination
普 济 消 毒 饮

■ **Ingredients**

Huang Qin	Scute	15g
Huang Lian	Coptis	15g
Chen Pi	Tangerine Peel	6g
Xuan Shen	Scrophularia	6g
Chai Hu	Bupleurum	6g
Jie Geng	Platycodon	6g
Lian Qiao	Forsythia Fruit	3g
Ban Lan Gen	Isatis Root	3g
Ma Bo	Lasiosphaera	3g
Niu Bang Zi	Burdock Seed	3g
Bo He	Peppermint	3g
Jiang Can	Bombyx	2g
Sheng Ma	Cimicifuga	2g
Gan Cao	Licorice	3g

■ **Preparation**
Use as decoction or prepared form.

■ **Pertaining Category**
Heat Clearing and Detoxicating

■ **Functions**
Clears heat, relieves toxicity. Expels wind-heat, benefits the throat.

■ **Indications**
Invasion of seasonal epidemic toxic heat with wind-heat manifested as high fever, chills, red, swelling head and face with burning pain, heavy eyes, sore throat, thirst, irritability, or mania, ulceration of mouth and tongue, constipation, dark and scanty urine, red and dry tongue with yellow coat, a rapid, forceful pulse.

■ **Cautions and Contraindications**

It is contraindicated in cases of Yin deficiency.

■ **Modern Applications**

Facial erysipelas, acute laryngopharyngitis, parotitis and tonsillitis, carbuncle, boils, and other skin infection on the head and face, herpes, etc.

Qi Bao Mei Ran Dan-Seven Treasure Elixir for Beautiful Whiskers

Fleece Flower Combination

七 宝 美 髯 丹

■ **Ingredients**

He Shou Wu	Fleece Flower Root	300g
Fu Ling	Hoelen/Poria	150g
Niu Xi	Achyranthes Root	150g
Dang Gui	Chinese Angelica	150g
Gou Qi Zi	Lycium Fruit	150g
Tu Si Zi	Dodder Seed	150g
Bu Gu Zhi	Scurfy Pea Fruit	120g

■ **Preparation**

Use as prepared form.

■ **Pertaining Category**

Yin Tonifying

■ **Functions**

Nourishes the kidney Yin and liver blood.

■ Indications

Yin deficiency of the kidney and liver with deficient liver blood manifested as early graying of the hair or hair loss, loose teeth, soreness and weakness of lower back and knees, nocturnal emission, spermatorrhea, pale tongue, a thin weak pulse.

■ Cautions and Contraindications

Use with caution for patients with indigestion due to spleen deficiency.

■ Modern Applications

Hair loss, baldness, premature graying hair, etc.

Qi Ju Di Huang Wan-Lycium, Chrysanthemum, and Rehmannia Pill
Lycium, Chrysanthemum, and Rehmannia Formula
杞 菊 地 黄 丸

■ Ingredients

Shu Di Huang	*Cooked Rehmannia*	24g
Shan Zhu Yu	*Dogwood Fruit*	12g
Shan Yao	*Dioscorea*	12g
Fu Ling	*Hoelen/Poria*	9g
Ze Xie	*Alisma*	9g
Mu Dan Pi	*Moutan Bark*	9g
Gou Qi Zi	*Lycium Fruit*	9g
Ju Hua	*Chrysanthemum*	9g

■ Preparation

Use as decoction or prepared form.

■ Pertaining Category

Yin Tonifying

■ Functions

Nourishes the liver and kidney Yin, brightens the eyes. Calms the liver Yang.

■ Indications

Yin deficiency of the liver and kidney with eye disturbances manifested as blurred and diminished vision, dry or painful eyes, tearing when exposed to wind, dizziness, vertigo, soreness and weakness of lower back, tinnitus, tidal fever, red tongue with scanty coat, a thin, rapid pulse.

■ Cautions and Contraindications

Use with extreme caution for patients with indigestion and diarrhea due to deficiency of the spleen and stomach.

■ Modern Applications

Diabetes, hypertension, arteriosclerosis, optic neuritis or atrophy, glaucoma, ophthalmalgia, retinitis, cataract, etc.

Qi Li San-Seven Thousandths of a Tael Powder
Musk and Catechu Formula
七厘散

■ Ingredients

Xue Jie	Dracaena	30g
She Xiang	Musk	0.4g
Bing Pian	Borneol	0.4g
Ru Xiang	Frankincense	5g
Mo Yao	Myrrh	5g
Hong Hua	Safflower	5g
Zhu Sha	Cinnabar	1-3g
Er Cha	Catechu	7.5g

Preparation
Use as fine powder internally or externally.

Pertaining Category
Blood Invigorating

Functions
Promotes blood circulation, dispels blood stasis, stops pain and bleeding.

Indications
External or internal injury due to trauma with blood stasis and strong constitution manifested as pain, bruises, bleeding, wounds, cuts, fracture, burns, scalds, as well as toxic swelling and pain.

Cautions and Contraindications
It is contraindicated during pregnancy. Do not use overdose and for long term.

Modern Applications
All kinds of external or internal traumatic injury.
Mix the powder with wine for external use.

Qian Zheng San-Pull Straight Powder
Lead to Symmetry Powder
牵 正 散

Ingredients

Bai Fu Zi	Typhonium	6g
Jiang Can	Bombyx	6g
Quan Xie	Scorpion	6g

Preparation
Use as decoction or prepared form.

Pertaining Category
External Wind Expelling

■ Functions
Expels wind, resolves phlegm, stops spasms.

■ Indications
Wind phlegm attacking the head and facial channels manifested as sudden deviation of mouth and eyes, muscle stiffness or spasms, or unable to close the eyes, swollen tongue with white greasy coat, a superficial or slippery pulse.

■ Cautions and Contraindications
This formula is toxic and should not be taken for long term. Do not use during pregnancy.

■ Modern Applications
Facial paralysis(Bell's palsy), trigeminal neuralgia, sequelae of cerebrovascular accident, etc.
It is inappropriate to use this formula alone for deviation of mouth and eyes due to endogenous liver wind with liver and kidney Yin deficiency.

Qiang Huo Sheng Shi Tang-Notopterygium Decoction to Overcome Dampness
Chianghuo and Vitex Combination
羌活胜湿汤

■ Ingredients

Qiang Huo	Notopterygium	6g
Du Huo	Tuhuo	6g
Gao Ben	Straw Weed	3g
Fang Feng	Siler	3g
Chuan Xiong	Ligusticum	3g
Man Jing Zi	Vitex Fruit	2g
Zhi Gan Cao	Baked Licorice	3g

Preparation
Use as decoction or prepared form.

Pertaining Category
Wind-dampness Expelling

Functions
Expels wind-dampness, releases the exterior, alleviates pain.

Indications
Wind-dampness invading the superficial channels manifested as heaviness and pain in the head, neck, shoulder, and back, difficulty in turning to side way, or general aching, slight chills and fever, lack of sweating, thin white tongue coat, a superficial, slow pulse.

Cautions and Contraindications
Use with caution for patients with Yin deficiency. It is contraindicated for patients with wind-heat invasion.

Modern Applications
Common cold, influenza, rheumatic arthritis, sciatica, etc.

Qin Jiao Bie Jia San-Gentiana Leaf and Tortoise Shell Powder
Chin-chiu and Turtle Shell Formula
秦艽鳖甲散

■ Ingredients

Qin Jiao	Big Leaf Gentiana	15g
Bie Jia	Tortoise Shell	30g
Di Gu Pi	Lycium Bark	30g
Chai Hu	Bupleurum	30g
Zhi Mu	Anemarrhena	15g
Dang Gui	Chinese Angelica	15g
Qing Hao	Sweet Wormwood	5 leaf
Wu Mei	Black Plum	1pc

■ Preparation
Use as prepared form or decoction with properly reduced dosage.

■ Pertaining Category
Deficient Heat Clearing

■ Functions
Nourishes Yin and blood, clears deficient heat, relieves steaming bone fever.

■ Indications
Invaded external pathogen turning to heat and hiding in the body with consumption of Yin manifested as steaming bone fever or afternoon fever, night sweats, emaciation, red cheeks and lips, lassitude, cough, dry mouth and throat, red tongue, a weak, rapid pulse.

■ Cautions and Contraindications
None noted.

■ Modern Applications
Pulmonary tuberculosis, anemia, chronic nephritis, fevers with unknown origin, post-surgical fever, chronic leukemia, malaria, and other chronic consumptive diseases, etc.

Qing Gu San-Clear the Bone-heat Powder
Cool the Bones Powder
清骨散

■ **Ingredients**

Yin Chai Hu	Stellaria Root	5g
Hu Huang Lian	Picrorhiza	3g
Qin Jiao	Big Leaf Gentiana	3g
Bie Jia	Tortoise Shell	3g
Di Gu Pi	Lycium Bark	3g
Qing Hao	Sweet Wormwood	3g
Zhi Mu	Anemarrhena	3g
Gan Cao	Licorice	2g

■ **Preparation**
Use as decoction or prepared form.

■ **Pertaining Category**
Deficient Heat Clearing

■ **Functions**
Clears deficient heat, reduces steaming bone heat.

■ **Indications**
Chronic consumptive disease with severe empty heat due to Yin deficiency manifested as tidal fever, lower graded fever, steaming bone fever, especially during afternoon or night, irritability, night sweats, malar flash, heat in the palms and soles, emaciation, dry mouth and throat, red tongue with scanty coat, a thin, rapid pulse.

■ **Cautions and Contraindications**
None noted.

■ **Modern Applications**
Pulmonary tuberculosis, bone tuberculosis, and other consumptive diseases, etc.

Qing Hao Bie Jia Tang-Sweet Wormwood and Turtoise Shell Decoction
Sweet Wormwood and Tortoise Shell Combination
青蒿鳖甲汤

■ Ingredients

Qing Hao	Sweet Wormwood	6g
Bie Jia	Tortoise Shell	15g
Sheng Di Huang	Dried Rehmannia	12g
Zhi Mu	Anemarrhena	6g
Mu Dan Pi	Moutan Bark	9g

■ Preparation
Use as decoction or prepared form.

■ Pertaining Category
Deficient Heat Clearing

■ Functions
Nourishes Yin, clears deficient heat.

■ Indications
Later stage of febrile disease with latent residual heat and Yin deficiency or chronic disease with damaged Yin manifested as lower grade fever at night and normal in the morning with absence of sweating as the fever subsides, emaciation, red tongue with scanty coat, a thin, rapid pulse.

■ Cautions and Contraindications
It is contraindicated in cases of tendency to convulsion due to Yin deficiency, or early stage of a warm-febrile disease when the pathogen is still in Wei and Qi levels.

■ Modern Applications
Pulmonary tuberculosis, anemia, chronic nephritis, fevers with unknown origin, post-surgical fever, chronic leukemia, malaria, and other chronic consumptive diseases, etc.

Qing Jin Hua Tan Tang-Clear Metal and Resolve Phlegm Decoction
清金化痰汤

■ **Ingredients**

Huang Qin	Scute	9g
Zhi Zi	Gardenia Fruit	6g
Jie Geng	Platycodon	6g
Mai Men Dong	Ophiopogon	9g
Sang Bai Pi	Mulberry Rootbark	9g
Zhe Bei Mu	Thunberg Fritillary	9g
Zhi Mu	Anemarrhena	9g
Gua Lou	Trichosanthes Fruit	6g
Chen Pi	Tangerine Peel	9g
Fu Ling	Hoelen/Poria	9g
Gan Cao	Licorice	6g

■ **Preparation**
Use as decoction or prepared form.

■ **Pertaining Category**
Heat Clearing and Phlegm Resolving

■ **Functions**
Clears the lung heat, resolves phlegm, stops coughing.

■ **Indications**
Phlegm-heat in the lungs with mild damage of the lung Yin
manifested as cough with excessive yellow, thick, and sticky
sputum that is difficult to expectorate, or bloody sputum, coarse
breathing, chest pain, red complexion, or fever, thirst, red tongue
with thin yellow coat, a slippery, rapid pulse.

■ **Cautions and Contraindications**
None noted.

■ **Modern Applications**
Acute or chronic bronchitis, pneumonia, asthma, etc.

247

Qing Jing San-Channel Clearing Powder
清 经 散

■ Ingredients

Mu Dan Pi	Moutan Bark	12g
Di Gu Pi	Lycium Rootbark	12g
Bai Shao Yao	White Peony	12g
Sheng Di Huang	Dried Rehmannia	12g
Qing Hao	Sweet Wormwood	9g
Huang Bai	Phellodendron Bar	9g
Fu Ling	Hoelen/Poria	6g

■ Preparation
Use as decoction or prepared form.

■ Pertaining Category
Additional Formulas for Ob-Gyn Disorders

■ Functions
Clears heat, cools blood, regulates menstruation.

■ Indications
Excess heat in the blood manifested as shortened menstrual cycle with excessive, dark red or purple colored, and thick sticky menstrual bleeding, irritability, a fullness and discomfort sensation in the chest, red complexion, dry mouth, dark and scanty urine, constipation, red tongue with yellow coat, a wiry, rapid pulse.

■ Cautions and Contraindications
None noted.

■ Modern Applications
Irregular menstruation, menorrhagia, polymenorrhea, etc.

Qing Luo Yin-Clear the Collaterals Beverage
Lotus Leaf and Lonicera Combination
清 络 饮

■ Ingredients

He Ye	Lotus Leaf	6g
Jin Yin Hua	Lonicera	6g
Si Gua Pi	Stringmelon Peel	6g
Xi Gua Cui Yi	Watermelon Peel	6g
Bian Dou Hua	Dolichos Flower	6g
Dan Zhu Ye	Bland Bamboo Leaf	6g

■ Preparation
Use as decoction.

■ Pertaining Category
Summer Heat Clearing

■ Functions
Expels and clears summer heat.

■ Indications
Mild summer heat invading Qi level and lungs manifested as fever, slight thirst, heavy and unclear head with blurred vision, or nausea, vomiting, and diarrhea, slight red tongue with thin white coat, a superficial, rapid pulse.

■ Cautions and Contraindications
None noted.

■ Modern Applications
Mild summer heat condition.

Qing Qi Hua Tan Wan-Clear Qi and Resolve Phlegm Pill
The Expectorant Pills
清气化痰丸

■ Ingredients

Gua Lou Ren	*Trichosanthes*	30g
Chen Pi	*Tangerine Peel*	30g
Huang Qin	*Scute*	30g
Xing Ren	*Apricot Seed*	30g
Zhi Shi	*Immature Citrus*	30g
Fu Ling	*Hoelen/Poria*	30g
Dan Nan Xing	*Arisaema Tuber*	45g
Ban Xia	*Pinellia Tuber*	45g

■ Preparation
Use as prepared form or decoction with properly reduced dosage.

■ Pertaining Category
Heat Clearing and Phlegm Resolving

■ Functions
Clears heat, resolves phlegm. Regulates and descends Qi, stops coughing.

■ Indications
Mild phlegm-heat in the lungs manifested as cough with yellow thick sticky sputum that is difficult to expectorate, a fullness and stifling sensation in the chest, or mild chest pain, nausea, dark and scanty urination, red tongue with yellow greasy coat, a slippery, rapid pulse.

■ Cautions and Contraindications
None noted.

■ Modern Applications
Acute or chronic bronchitis, pneumonia, etc.

Qing Re Gu Jing Tang-Clear Heat and Secure Menses Decoction
清 热 固 经 汤

■ Ingredients

Huang Qin	*Scute*	9g
Jiao Zhi Zi	*Charred Gardenia*	9g
Sheng Di Huang	*Dried Rehmannia*	12g
Di Gu Pi	*Lycium Rootbark*	12g
Di Yu	*Sanguisorba Root*	9g
E Jiao	*Equus/Gelatin*	9g
Ou Jie	*Lotus Node*	9g
Zong Lu Tan	*Trachycarpus*	9g
Gui Ban	*Tortoise Plastron*	15g
Mu Li	*Oyster Shell*	15g
Gan Cao	*Licorice*	6g

■ Preparation
Use as decoction or prepared form. E Jiao should be dissolved in boiling water and added into the strained decoction.

■ Pertaining Category
Additional Formulas for Ob-Gyn Disorders

■ Functions
Clears heat, cools blood, stops bleeding. Regulates menstruation.

■ Indications
Excess heat in the blood leading to sudden, severe, heavy uterine bleeding with deep bright red colored blood and thick quality, thirst, irritability, or fever, dark and scanty urine, dry stools, red tongue with yellow or yellow greasy coat, rapid, forceful pulse.

■ Cautions and Contraindications
None noted.

■ Modern Applications
Uterine bleeding, menorrhagia, etc.

Qing Shu Yi Qi Tang-Clear Summer Heat and Tonify Qi Decoction

Lotus Stem and Ginseng Combination

清暑益气汤

■ **Ingredients**

Xi Yang Shen	American Ginseng	5g
Shi Hu	Dendrobium	15g
Mai Men Dong	Ophiopogon	9g
Huang Lian	Coptis	3g
Dan Zhu Ye	Bland Bamboo Leaf	6g
He Geng	Lotus Stem	15g
Zhi Mu	Anemarrhena	6g
Gan Cao	Licorice	3g
Geng Mi	Oryza	15g
Xi Gua Cui Yi	Watermelon Peel	30g

■ **Preparation**

Use as decoction or prepared form.

■ **Pertaining Category**

Summer Heat Clearing

■ **Functions**

Clears summer heat, eliminates dampness. Tonifies Qi. Nourishes Yin, promotes the generation of body fluid.

■ **Indications**

Summer heat with consumption of Qi and Yin manifested as fever, profuse sweating, irritability, thirst, dark and scanty urine, lassitude, shortness of breath, listlessness, red tongue, a feeble, rapid pulse.

■ **Cautions and Contraindications**

None noted.

■ **Modern Applications**

Common cold in the summer, sunstroke, heat stroke, summer fever in children, etc.

This formula is from " *Wen Re Jing Wei* "*(Warp and Woof of Warm-febrile Disease).*

Qing Wei San-Clear the Stomach Powder
Coptis and Rehmannia Formula
清胃散

■ **Ingredients**

Sheng Di Huang	Dried Rehmannia	12g
Dang Gui	Chinese Angelica	6g
Huang Lian	Coptis	3-5g
Mu Dan Pi	Moutan Bark	9g
Sheng Ma	Cimicifuga	6g

■ **Preparation**
Use as decoction or prepared form.

■ **Pertaining Category**
Clearing Heat from Zang-fu Organs

■ **Functions**
Clears the stomach heat, cools blood.

■ **Indications**
Heat in the stomach manifested as toothache, headache, bleeding, swelling, or ulcerated gums, feverish cheeks, aversion to heat, thirst with a desire to drink cold water, swelling and pain of lips and cheek, dry mouth, bad breath, red and dry tongue with yellow coat, a slippery, rapid, and forceful pulse.

■ **Cautions and Contraindications**
It is contraindicated in cases of toothache due to wind-cold invasion or Yin deficiency.

■ **Modern Applications**
Toothache, stomatitis, gingivitis, periodontitis, glossitis, trigeminal neuralgia, idiopathic halitosis, thrombocytopenic purpura, etc.

Qing Wen Bai Du Yin-Clear Epidemics and Antitoxin Beverage

Gypsum and Rhinoceros Horn Combination

清瘟敗毒飲

■ **Ingredients**

Shi Gao	Gypsum	30-60g
Sheng Di Huang	Dried Rehmannia	15g
Xi Jiao	Rhinoceros Horn	3g
Huang Lian	Coptis	6g
Zhi Zi	Gardenia Fruit	6g
Huang Qin	Scute	6g
Jie Geng	Platycodon	3g
Zhi Mu	Anemarrhena	6g
Chi Shao Yao	Red Peony	6g
Xuan Shen	Scrophularia	6g
Lian Qiao	Forsythia Fruit	6g
Mu Dan Pi	Moutan Bark	6g
Dan Zhu Ye	Bland Bamboo Leaf	3g
Gan Cao	Licorice	3g

■ **Preparation**

Use as decoction or prepared form. Shi Gao should be decocted first; Xi Jiao should be ground into powder and taken with the decoction; Xi Jiao may be substituted by Shui Niu Jiao (Horn of Water Buffalo) with a dosage of 30-120g.

■ **Pertaining Category**

Qi and Blood Level Heat Clearing

■ **Functions**

Clears heat from Qi level, relieves toxicity. Cools blood, stops bleeding. Nourishes Yin.

254

Indications

Intense epidemic toxic heat in both Qi and blood level manifested as high fever, thirst, severe headache, retching, irritability, delirium, or coma, or vomiting of blood, nosebleeding, skin rashes, or convulsion, or cold extremities, dark red tongue with cracked lips, a deep, thin, and rapid pulse or superficial, rapid pulse.

Cautions and Contraindications

This formula is extremely cold and should not be used for patients without exuberant and toxic heat.

Modern Applications

Severe influenza, encephalitis B, epidemic cerebrospinal meningitis, septicemia, erysipelas, etc.

Qing Xin Lian Zi Yin-Clear the Heart Beverage with Lotus Seed
Lotus Seed Combination
清 心 莲 子 饮

Ingredients

Huang Qin	Scute	6-9g
Mai Men Dong	Ophiopogon	6-9g
Di Gu Pi	Lycium Bark	6-9g
Che Qian Zi	Plantago Seed	6-9g
Lian Zi	Lotus Seed	6-9g
Fu Ling	Hoelen/Poria	6-9g
Huang Qi	Astragalus	6-9g
Ren Shen	Ginseng	6-9g
Zhi Gan Cao	Baked Licorice	3-6g

Preparation

Use as decoction or prepared form.

■ Pertaining Category
Clearing Heat from Zang-fu Organs

■ Functions
Clears heart fire, relieves urinary strangury. Tonifies Qi and Yin.

■ Indications
Heart fire and lower burner damp-heat with Qi and Yin deficiency manifested as dark and difficult urination, yellow leukorrhea, nocturnal emission, uterine bleeding, all of which is aggravated by over exertion, dryness or ulceration of mouth and tongue, irritability, or insomnia, fever, red face, thirst, red tongue with yellow greasy coat, or no coat, a thin, rapid pulse.

■ Cautions and Contraindications
None noted.

■ Modern Applications
Chronic UTI, chronic cystitis, chronic pyelonephritis, chronic prostatitis, leukorrhea, uterine bleeding, etc.

Qing Ying Tang-Clear the Nutritive Level Decoction
Rhinoceros and Scrophularia Combination
清营汤

■ Ingredients

Xi Jiao	Rhinoceros Horn	3g
Sheng Di Huang	Dried Rehmannia	15g
Xuan Shen	Scrophularia	9g
Dan Zhu Ye	Bland Bamboo Leaf	3g
Mai Men Dong	Ophiopogon	9g
Dan Shen	Salvia Root	6g
Huang Lian	Coptis	5g
Jin Yin Hua	Lonicera	9g
Lian Qiao	Forsythia	6g

■ Preparation
Use as decoction or prepared form. Xi Jiao should be taken in powder form with strained decoction; it may be substituted by Shui Niu Jiao (Horn of the Water Buffalo) with 30g in decoction or 6g as a powder; it should be decocted separately for 15-20 minutes prior to other ingredients.

■ Pertaining Category
Yin and Blood Level Cooling

■ Functions
Clears heat from nutritive level, relieves toxicity. Nourishes Yin, promotes blood circulation.

■ Indications
Heat penetrating into Ying (Nutritive level) manifested as feverish body, especially at night, irritability, insomnia, occasional delirium, faint skin rashes or macula, thirst or no thirst, dark red and dry tongue, a thin, rapid pulse.

■ Cautions and Contraindications
It is contraindicated in cases of dampness retention with white moist tongue coat.

■ Modern Applications
Severe influenza, encephalitis B, epidemic meningitis, septicemia, scarlet fever, erysipelas, etc.

257

Qing Zao Jiu Fei Tang-Clear Dryness and Rescue the Lung Decoction
Eriobotrya and Ophiopogon Combination
清燥救肺汤

■ **Ingredients**

Sang Ye	Mulberry Leaf	9g
Shi Gao	Gypsum	7.5g
Ren Shen	Ginseng	2g
Hei Zhi Ma	Sesame Seed	3g
E Jiao	Equus/Gelatin	2.4g
Mai Men Dong	Ophiopogon	3.6g
Xing Ren	Apricot Seed	2g
Pi Pa Ye	Eriobotrya Leaf	3g
Gan Cao	Licorice	3g

■ **Preparation**
Use as decoction or prepared form. E Jiao should be dissolved separately in boiling water and added into strained decoction.

■ **Pertaining Category**
Moistening Dryness

■ **Functions**
Clears dry-heat, moistens the lung Yin.

■ **Indications**
Dry-heat attacking the lungs with damage of the lung Yin and mild injury of lung Qi manifested as headache, feverish body, dry cough with no sputum, dyspnea, dry throat and nose, fullness of chest, pain in the hypochondrium, irritability, thirst, pink tongue with dry scanty coat or no coat, a feeble, thin, and rapid pulse.

■ Cautions and Contraindications

Use with caution for patients with weakness of the spleen and stomach. It should not be used for deficient pattern without excess heat unless it is modified.

■ Modern Applications

Pharyngitis, bronchitis, bronchiectasis, pneumonia, pulmonary tuberculosis, asthma, etc.

Ren Shen Bai Du San-Ginseng Overcome Toxicity Powder

Ginseng and Mentha Formula
人参败毒散

■ Ingredients

Chai Hu	Bupleurum	30g
Qian Hu	Hogfennel Root	30g
Chuan Xiong	Ligusticum	30g
Zhi Ke	Bitter Orange	30g
Qiang Huo	Notopterygium	30g
Du Huo	Tuhuo	30g
Fu Ling	Hoelen/Poria	30g
Jie Geng	Platycodon	30g
Ren Shen	Ginseng	30g
Gan Cao	Licorice	15g
Sheng Jiang	Fresh Ginger	9g
Bo He	Peppermint	6g

■ Preparation

Use as prepared form or decoction with properly reduced dosage.

■ Pertaining Category

Strengthening Body Resistance and Relieving Exterior

■ **Functions**
Expels wind-cold-dampness, releases the exterior. Tonifies Qi.
Resolves phlegm.

■ **Indications**
Invasion of wind-cold-dampness with weakened body resistance
manifested as aversion to wind-cold, fever, headache, stiffness neck,
soreness and heaviness of the body and limbs, absence of sweating,
stuffy nose, fullness in the chest, cough with white sputum, white
greasy tongue coat, a superficial, soft pulse which turns weak on
harder pressure.

■ **Cautions and Contraindications**
It is contraindicated in cases of damp-heat retention, because this
formula is warm and dry.

■ **Modern Applications**
Common cold, influenza, malaria, suppurative infection, dysentery,
epidemic parotitis, urticaria, eczema, measles, rheumatic arthritis,
etc.
*This formula is also known as Bai Du San (Overcome Toxicity
Powder).*

Ren Shen Ge Jie San-Ginseng and Gecko
Powder
Ginseng and Gecko Combination
人 参 蛤 蚧 散

■ Ingredients

Ren Shen	Ginseng	60g
Ge Jie	Gecko	1pair
Fu Ling	Hoelen/Poria	60g
Chuan Bei Mu	Tendrilled Fritillary	60g
Xing Ren	Apricot Seed	150g
Sang Bai Pi	Morus Rootbark	60g
Zhi Mu	Anemarrhena	60g
Zhi Gan Cao	Baked Licorice	150g

■ Preparation
Use as prepared form.

■ Pertaining Category
Qi Tonifying

■ Functions
Tonifies the lung Qi. Clears the lung heat, resolves phlegm, stops cough and asthma.

■ Indications
Lung, spleen, and kidney Qi deficiency with phlegm-damp and slight heat manifested as chronic cough, difficulty in breathing, yellow, sticky sputum or coughing of bloody pus, irritable heat in the chest, emaciation, or facial and body edema, thin white or thin yellow greasy tongue coat, a superficial, weak pulse.

■ Cautions and Contraindications
It is contraindicated in cases of cough or asthma in exterior and excess patterns.

■ Modern Applications
Chronic bronchitis, chronic bronchial asthma, emphysema, pulmonary tuberculosis, lung abscess, etc.

Ren Shen Hu Tao Tang-Ginseng and Walnut Decoction

Ginseng and Walnut Combination
人参胡桃汤

■ Ingredients

Ren Shen	Ginseng	6-9g
Hu Tao Ren	Walnut	5pcs
Sheng Jiang	Fresh Ginger	5slices

■ Preparation
Use as decoction or prepared form.

■ Pertaining Category
Qi Tonifying

■ Functions
Tonifies the lung and kidney Qi, stops wheezing and coughing.

■ Indications
Lung and kidney Qi deficiency with inability to grasp Qi manifested as coughing, wheezing, shortness of breath, low voice, soreness and weakness of lower back, slight aversion to cold, cold hands and feet, pale tongue with thin white coat, a weak, feeble pulse.

■ Cautions and Contraindications
None noted.

■ Modern Applications
Chronic bronchitis, chronic bronchial asthma, pulmonary emphysema, etc.

Ren Shen Yang Rong Tang-Ginseng Nourish Nutritive Qi Decoction

Ginseng Nutritive Combination
人参养荣汤

Ingredients

Ren Shen	Ginseng	6-9g
Bai Zhu	White Atractylodes	9-12g
Fu Ling	Hoelen/Poria	9-12g
Shu Di Huang	Cooked Rehmannia	9-12g
Bai Shao Yao	White Peony	9-12g
Dang Gui	Chinese Angelica	9-12g
Huang Qi	Astragalus	9-12g
Rou Gui	Cinnamon Bark	3-6g
Chen Pi	Tangerine Peel	3-6g
Yuan Zhi	Polygala	6-9g
Wu Wei Zi	Schizandra	6-9g
Zhi Gan Cao	Baked Licorice	3-6g
Sheng Jiang	Fresh Ginger	3slices
Da Zao	Jujube	2pcs

■ Preparation
Use as decoction or prepared form.

■ Pertaining Category
Qi and Blood Tonifying

■ Functions
Tonifies Qi and blood, nourishes the heart, calms spirit.

■ Indications
Consumptive diseases with the lung and spleen Qi, heart blood, and Yang deficiency with disturbance of spirit manifested as shortness of breath that is worse on exertion, palpitation, insomnia, forgetfulness, pale and lusterless complexion, dry throat and lips, emaciation, loss of appetite, or amenorrhea, pale tongue with thin white coat, a thin, weak pulse.

Cautions and Contraindications
None noted.

Modern Applications
Anemia, postpartum recovery, neurasthenia, amenorrhea, insomnia, pulmonary tuberculosis, optic atrophy, chronic non-healing ulcers, etc

Run Chang Wan-Moisten the Intestine Pill
The Emollient Pills
润 肠 丸

■ Ingredients

Huo Ma Ren	Hemp Seed	9-15g
Tao Ren	Peach Kernel	6-9g
Dang Gui	Chinese Angelica	9-12g
Sheng Di Huang	Dried Rehmannia	9-15g
Zhi Ke	Bitter Orange	6-9g

■ Preparation
Use as prepared form or decoction

■ Pertaining Category
Purging Downward with Moist Laxatives

■ Functions
Moistens the intestines, moves the bowels. Nourishes Yin and blood.

■ Indications
Dryness of the intestines due to Yin or blood deficiency manifested as constipation, lusterless complexion and nails, dry skin and mouth, or dizziness, palpitation, pale or dry tongue, a thin pulse.

■ **Cautions and Contraindications**
None noted.

■ **Modern Applications**
Habitual constipation, postpartum or post-surgical constipation, hemorrhoids, anal fissure, etc.
This formula is from "Shen Shi Zun Sheng Shu" (Master Shen's Book for Revering Life).

San Ao Tang-Three Stubborn Decoction
Ma Huang, Apricot Seed, and licorice Combination
三 拗 汤

■ **Ingredients**

Ma Huang	Ephedra	5g
Xing Ren	Apricot Seed	5g
Gan Cao	Licorice	5g
Sheng Jiang	Fresh Ginger	5slices

■ **Preparation**
Use as decoction or prepared form.

■ **Pertaining Category**
Pungent Warm Exterior Relieving

■ **Functions**
Opens the lungs, relieves asthma. Expels wind-cold, releases the exterior.

■ **Indications**
Mild exterior wind-cold invasion affecting the lungs manifested as aversion to wind-cold, headache and body aches, nasal congestion, heavy sensation in the body, loss of voice, cough with excessive white sputum, fullness in the chest, shortness of breath, thin white tongue coat, a superficial, tight pulse.

Cautions and Contraindications

It is contraindicated in cases of exterior wind-heat, exterior deficiency, and weak constitution. Use with caution for patients with hypertension and heart problems.

Modern Applications

Bronchitis, bronchial asthma, pneumonia, whooping cough, etc. *This formula is modified from Ma Huang Tang (Ephedra Decoction).*

San Bi Tang-Three Painful Obstruction Decoction
Teasel and Eucommia Combination
三痹汤

Ingredients

Xu Duan	*Teasel Root*	5g
Du Zhong	*Eucommia Bark*	5g
Fang Feng	*Siler*	5g
Rou Gui	*Cinnamon Bark*	5g
Xi Xin	*Asarum*	3g
Ren Shen	*Ginseng*	5g
Fu Ling	*Hoelen/Poria*	5g
Dang Gui	*Chinese Angelica*	5g
Bai Shao Yao	*White Peony*	5g
Huang Qi	*Astragalus*	5g
Niu Xi	*Achyranthes Root*	5g
Qin Jiao	*Big Leaf Gentiana*	3g
Sheng Di Huang	*Dried Rehmannia*	3g
Chuan Xiong	*Ligusticum*	3g
Du Huo	*Tuhuo*	3g
Sheng Jiang	*Fresh Ginger*	3g
Gan Cao	*Licorice*	5g

■   **Preparation**
Use as decoction or prepared form.

■   **Pertaining Category**
Wind-dampness Expelling

■   **Functions**
Tonifies Qi and blood, nourishes the liver and kidney, strengthens tendons and bones. Expels wind-dampness.

■   **Indications**
Chronic bi syndrome due to wind-dampness invasion with Qi and blood deficiency and weakness of the liver and kidney manifested as pain, heaviness, and coldness of lower back and knees, preference to warmth and aversion to damp-cold, weakness and numbness of limbs, or tremors and spasms in the extremities, pale tongue with white coat, a deep, weak pulse.

■   **Cautions and Contraindications**
Xi Xin (Asarum) can not be used overdose or for a long term.

■   **Modern Applications**
Chronic osteoarthritis, lumbago, sciatica, chronic rheumatic or rheumatoid arthritis, sequelae of poliomyelitis, etc.

San Cai Feng Sui Dan-Three-talent Retainin Marrow Elixir
Heaven, Human, and Earth Marrow Retaining Formula
三 才 封 髓 丹

- **Ingredients**

Shu Di Huang	Cooked Rehmannia	24g
Tian Men Dong	Asparagus	9g
Ren Shen	Ginseng	9g
Huang Bai	Phellodendron	9g
Sha Ren	Amomum Fruit	3g
Gan Cao	Licorice	6g

- **Preparation**

Use as decoction or prepared form.

- **Pertaining Category**

Additional Formulas for Internal Medicine

- **Functions**

Nourishes the kidney Yin, clears the heart fire. Calms spirit, secures essence.

- **Indications**

Kidney Yin deficiency with exuberant empty fire manifested as insomnia, dream disturbed sleep, nocturnal emission, irritable heat in the chest, palpitation, dry mouth, dizziness, vertigo, lassitude, forgetfulness, night sweats, soreness and weakness of lower back and knees, dark and scanty urine, red tongue with little coat, a thin, rapid pulse.

- **Cautions and Contraindications**

None noted.

- **Modern Applications**

Seminal emission, chronic nephritis, diabetes, menopausal syndrome, neurasthenia, etc.

San Jia Fu Mai Tang-Three Shell Decoction to Restore the Pulse

Decoction of Three Shells to Recover the Pulse

三甲复脉汤

■ Ingredients

Zhi Gan Cao	Baked Licorice	18g
Sheng Di Huang	Dried Rehmannia	18g
Bai Shao Yao	White Peony	18g
Mai Men Dong	Ophiopogon	15g
E Jiao	Equus/Gelatin	9g
Mu Li	Oyster Shell	15g
Bie Jia	Tortoise Shell	24g
Gui Ban	Tortoise Plastron	30g
Huo Ma Ren	Hemp Seed	10g

■ Preparation
Use as decoction or prepared form. E Jiao should be dissolved separately in boiling water and added into the strained decoction. Bie Jia, Mu Li, and Gui Ban should be crushed and cooked 45 minutes prior to the other herbs.

■ Pertaining Category
Internal Wind Extinguishing

■ Functions
Nourishes Yin, restores the pulse. Suppresses Yang, extinguishes wind.

■ Indications
Endogenous wind or liver Yang raising due to Yin and blood deficiency in the later stage of febrile disease or from internal disorders manifested as spasms of the muscles, trembling of hands, severe palpitation, or chest pain, a heat sensation in the palms and soles, dizziness, vertigo, tinnitus, dry throat, dark red and dry tongue with scanty coat, a thin, rapid pulse.

■ Cautions and Contraindications

Use with extreme caution during pregnancy and for patients with diarrhea due to weakness of the spleen and stomach.

■ Modern Applications

Chronic convulsion, Parkinson's disease, encephalitis, meningitis, hypocalcemia, anemia, tinnitus, vertigo, etc.

San Miao Wan (San)-Three Mysterious Pill(Powder)
Three Marvel Pill (Powder)
三 妙 丸 (散)

■ Ingredients

Huang Bai	Phellodendron	120g
Cang Zhu	Atractylodes	180g
Chuan Niu Xi	Cyathula Root	60g

■ Preparation

Use as prepared form or decoction with properly reduced dosage.

■ Pertaining Category

Damp-heat Clearing

■ Functions

Clears heat, dries dampness. Invigorates blood circulation.

■ Indications

Damp-heat in the lower burner manifested as lower back pain, red, hot, swollen knees and feet with burning pain, numbness of feet, weakness of lower back and lower limbs, yellow and odorous vaginal discharge, dark, yellow, and scanty urine, red tongue with yellow greasy coat, a slippery, rapid pulse.

- **Cautions and Contraindications**

None noted.

- **Modern Applications**

Acute or chronic UTI, vaginitis, cervicitis, rheumatic, rheumatoid, or gouty arthritis, beriberi, etc.

San Ren Tang-Three Seeds Decoction
Apricot, Coix, and Cluster Combination
三仁汤

- **Ingredients**

Xing Ren	Apricot Seed	15g
Yi Yi Ren	Coix Seed	18g
Bai Dou Kou	Cluster	6g
Hua Shi	Talcum	18g
Tong Cao	Rice Paper Pith	6g
Dan Zhu Ye	Bland Bamboo Leaf	6g
Ban Xia	Pinellia Tuber	9g
Hou Po	Magnolia Bark	6g

- **Preparation**

Use as decoction or prepared form.

- **Pertaining Category**

Damp-heat Clearing

- **Functions**

Promotes the movement of Qi, clears heat, drains dampness.

- **Indications**

External or internal damp-heat (damp is more predominant) obstructing in the Qi level manifested as headache, chills, fever in the afternoon, aching and heaviness of the body, slight yellow complexion, a stifling sensation in the chest, loss of appetite, absence of thirst, white tongue coat, a wiry, thin, and soft pulse.

■ **Cautions and Contraindications**

It is contraindicated in cases of deficiency of Yin, blood, and body fluids. Use cautiously for damp-heat condition with pronounced heat.

■ **Modern Applications**

Acute gastroenteritis, influenza, acute hepatitis, acute pyelonephritis, etc.

San Wu Bei Ji Wan-Three Substances for Emergency Pill
Rhubarb, Ginger, and Croton Formula
三物备急丸

■ **Ingredients**

Da Huang	*Rhubarb*	30g
Gan Jiang	*Dried Ginger*	30g
Ba Dou	*Croton Seed*	30g

■ **Preparation**

Use as powder or pill form (made with honey).

■ **Pertaining Category**

Purging Downward with Warm Nature

■ **Functions**

Vigorously purges cold accumulation.

■ **Indications**

Sudden severe interior excess cold accumulation manifested as epigastric and abdominal severe pricky pain, rough, uneven breathing, constipation, blue-purple tongue with white coat, a deep, tight pulse. In severe cases, there may also be loss of consciousness with lockjaw.

■ Cautions and Contraindications

Ba Dou (Croton Seed) is pungent, hot, and very toxic, it should be used with extreme caution. It is contraindicated in cases of pregnant woman, elderly, and patients with weak constitution.

■ Modern Applications

Intestinal obstruction without complication, food poisoning, acute pancreatitis, and uncomplicated appendicitis, etc.

San Zi Yang Qin Tang-Three Seeds Nourishing the Parents Decoction
Three-seed Decoction to Nourish One's Parents
三子养亲汤

■ Ingredients

Bai Jie Zi	Brassica Seed	6g
Zi Su Zi	Perilla Seed	9g
Lai Fu Zi	Radish Seed	9g

■ Preparation

Use as decoction or prepared form.

■ Pertaining Category

Cold-phlegm Transforming

■ Functions

Descends Qi, relieves discomfort in the chest and diaphragm. Resolves phlegm, promotes digestion.

■ Indications

Cold-phlegm in the lungs with Qi and food stagnation manifested as cough and wheezing with profuse white sputum, a stifling sensation in the chest, poor appetite and indigestion, white greasy tongue coat, a slippery pulse.

Cautions and Contraindications
The cause of disease should be treated once the effects are obtained.

Modern Applications
Chronic bronchitis, bronchial asthma, pulmonary emphysema, bronchiectasis, etc.

Sang Bai Pi Tang-Mulberry Rootbark Decoction
Mulberry Rootbark Combination
桑白皮汤

Ingredients

Sang Bai Pi	*Mulberry Rootbark*	12g
Ban Xia	*Pinellia Tuber*	9g
Zi Su Zi	*Perilla Seed*	9g
Xing Ren	*Apricot Seed*	9g
Zhe Bei Mu	*Thunberg Fritillary*	9g
Huang Qin	*Scute*	9g
Huang Lian	*Coptis*	6g
Zhi Zi	*Gardenia fruit*	9g

Preparation
Use as decoction or prepared form.

Pertaining Category
Heat Clearing and Phlegm Resolving

Functions
Clears the lung heat, resolves phlegm, relieves coughing and wheezing.

274

■ Indications

Phlegm-heat in the lungs manifested as cough and wheezing with yellow, thick, sticky, or bloody sputum, distending pain in the chest with irritable heat sensation, feverish body, sweats, thirst with a desire for cold drink, red complexion, dry throat, dark and scanty urine, or constipation, red tongue with yellow greasy coat, a slippery, rapid pulse.

■ Cautions and Contraindications

Use cautiously for patients with significant spleen and stomach deficiency.

■ Modern Applications

Acute or chronic bronchitis, pneumonia, asthma, etc.

Sang Ju Yin-Mulberry Leaf and Chrysanthemum Beverage
Morus and Chrysanthemum Combination
桑 菊 饮

■ Ingredients

Sang Ye	*Mulberry Leaf*	7.5g
Ju Hua	*Chrysanthemum*	3g
Xing Ren	*Apricot Seed*	6g
Lian Qiao	*Forsythia Fruit*	5g
Bo He	*Peppermint*	2.5g
Jie Geng	*Platycodon*	6g
Lu Gen	*Reed Rhizome*	6g
Gan Cao	*Licorice*	2.5g

■ Preparation

Use as decoction or prepared form. Do not cook for more than 20 minutes. Bo He should be added 5 minutes near the end of cooking.

■ Pertaining Category

Pungent Cool Exterior Relieving

■ Functions

Expels wind-heat, releases the exterior. Disperses the lung Qi, stops coughing.

■ Indications

Early stage of wind-heat invasion marked by cough, slight chills, or fever, thirst, thin white or yellowish tongue coat, a superficial, rapid pulse.

■ Cautions and Contraindications

It is contraindicated in cases of cough due to wind-cold invasion.

■ Modern Applications

Common cold, influenza, acute laryngopharyngitis, acute tonsillitis, acute bronchitis, acute conjunctivitis, etc.

Sang Piao Xiao San-Praying Mantis Egg-case Powder
Mantis Formula
桑螵蛸散

■ Ingredients

Sang Piao Xiao	*Mantis Egg-case*	30g
Yuan Zhi	*Polygala*	30g
Shi Chang Pu	*Sweetflag Rhizome*	30g
Long Gu	*Dragon Bone*	30g
Ren Shen	*Ginseng*	30g
Fu Shen	*Hoelen/Poria*	30g
Dang Gui	*Chinese Angelica*	30g
Gui Ban	*Tortoise Plastron*	30g

■ **Preparation**
Use as prepared form or decoction with properly reduced dosage.

■ **Pertaining Category**
Binding the Essence to Stop Seminal Emission and Enuresis

■ **Functions**
Tonifies and regulates the heart and kidney, consolidares essence.

■ **Indications**
Qi and Yin deficiency of the heart and kidney with disharmony and spirit disturbance manifested as frequent or cloudy urination, or even incontinence of urine, enuresis, or spermatorrhea, palpitation, absentmindedness, poor memory, dream disturbed sleep, or poor appetite, pale or red tongue with thin white coat, a thin, weak pulse.

■ **Cautions and Contraindications**
It is contraindicated in cases of frequent urination, enuresis, or seminal emission caused by damp-heat in the lower burner.

■ **Modern Applications**
Enuresis, neurasthenia, diabetes, dysfunction of endocrine system, seminal emission, sexual dysfunction, etc.

Sang Xing Tang-Morus and Apricot Seed Decoction
Morus and Apricot Seed Combination
桑 杏 汤

■ Ingredients

Sang Ye	Mulberry Leaf	3g
Xing Ren	Apricot Seed	4.5g
Sha Shen	Glehnia Root	6g
Zhe Bei Mu	Thunberg Fritillary	3g
Dan Dou Chi	Prepared Soybean	3g
Zhi Zi	Gardenia Fruit	3g
Li Pi	Pear Peel	3g

■ Preparation
Use as decoction or prepared form.

■ Pertaining Category
Moistening Dryness

■ Functions
Gently expels wind-heat and dryness, moistens the lungs, stops coughing.

■ Indications
External wind-heat and dryness attacking the lungs manifested as headache, fever, thirst, cough with no sputum or scanty sticky sputum that is hard to expectorate, dry throat, red tongue with dry, thin white coat, a superficial, rapid pulse.

■ Cautions and Contraindications
It is contraindicated in cases of cough due to wind-cold or phlegm-cold.

■ Modern Applications
Common cold, pharyngitis, acute bronchitis, upper respiratory infection, bronchiectasis, etc.

Sha Shen Mai Men Dong Tang-Glehnia and Ophiopogon Decoction

Adenophora and Ophiopogon Combination

沙参麦门冬汤

■ Ingredients

Sha Shen	Glehnia Root	9g
Mai Men Dong	Ophiopogon	9g
Yu Zhu	Polygonatum	6g
Sang Ye	Mulberry Leaf	4.5g
Bian Dou	Dolichos	4.5g
Tian Hua Fen	Trichosanthes Root	4.5g
Gan Cao	Licorice	3g

■ Preparation
Use as decoction or prepared form.

■ Pertaining Category
Moistening Dryness

■ Functions
Nourishes the lung and stomach Yin, generates body fluid, moistens dryness.

■ Indications
Lung and stomach Yin deficiency due to dry-heat manifested as dry throat, thirst, or slight fever, dry cough with scanty sputum or no sputum, red and dry tongue with scanty coat, a thin, weak, and rapid pulse.

■ Cautions and Contraindications
None noted.

■ Modern Applications
Pharyngitis, bronchitis, bronchiectasis, pulmonary tuberculosis, chronic gastritis, etc.

Shao Fu Zhu Yu Tang-Remove Blood Stasis in the Lower Abdomen Decoction
Cnidium and Bulrush Combination
少 腹 逐 瘀 汤

■ **Ingredients**

Xiao Hui Xiang	Fennel Fruit	1.5g
Gan Jiang	Dried Ginger	0.6-3g
Yan Hu Suo	Corydalis	3g
Dang Gui	Chinese Angelica	9g
Chuan Xiong	Ligusticum	3g
Rou Gui	Cinnamon Bark	3g
Mo Yao	Myrrh	3g
Chi Shao Yao	Red Peony	6g
Pu Huang	Cattail Pollen	9g
Wu Ling Zhi	Trogopterus	6g

■ **Preparation**
Use as decoction or prepared form. Wu Ling Zhi should be wrapped in gauze when making decoction.

■ **Pertaining Category**
Blood Invigorating

■ **Functions**
Promotes blood circulation, removes blood stasis. Warms channels, stops pain.

■ **Indications**
Blood stasis in the lower burner due to cold manifested as mass in the lower abdomen with or without pain, or pain and distention in the lower abdomen without mass, soreness of lower back and abdominal bloating during menstruation, dark menses or uterine bleeding with clots and lower lateral abdominal pain, purple tongue, a wiry, hesitant pulse.

■ **Cautions and Contraindications**

It is contraindicated during pregnancy and in cases of excessive menstrual bleeding, bleeding diathesis, or any bleeding disorders, etc.

■ **Modern Applications**

Dysmenorrhea, amenorrhea, irregular menstruation, abdominal mass uterus fibroids, uterine bleeding, cirrhosis of liver, etc.

Shao Yao Gan Cao Tang-Peony and Licorice Decoction
Peony and Licorice Combination
芍 药 甘 草 汤

■ **Ingredients**

Bai Shao Yao	White Peony	12g
Zhi Gan Cao	Baked Licorice	12g

■ **Preparation**

Use as decoction or prepared form.

■ **Pertaining Category**

Regulating the Liver and Spleen(Mediating)

■ **Functions**

Soothes the liver, relieves spasms, stops pain.

■ **Indications**

Disharmony between the liver and spleen or blood and Yin deficiency with poor circulation manifested as spasmodic abdominal pain, irritability, cramping pain in the calf muscles or hands, red or pale tongue with scanty coat, a thin, weak, or wiry pulse.

■ Cautions and Contraindications
None noted.

■ Modern Applications
Dysfunction of stomach and intestines, intercostal neuralgia,
trigeminal neuralgia, sciatica, primary dysmenorrhea, frozen
shoulder, etc.

Shao Yao Tang-Peony Decoction
Peony Combination
芍 药 汤

■ Ingredients

Bai Shao Yao	White Peony	15g
Dang Gui	Chinese Angelica	9g
Huang Lian	Coptis	9g
Bing Lang	Betel Nut	5g
Mu Xiang	Saussurea	5g
Huang Qin	Scute	9g
Da Huang	Rhubarb	9g
Rou Gui	Cinnamon Bark	5g
Gan Cao	Licorice	5g

■ Preparation
Use as decoction or prepared form.

■ Pertaining Category
Clearing Heat from Zang-fu Organs

■ Functions
Clears damp-heat, relieves toxicity. Regulates Qi and blood.

■ Indications
Damp-heat in the large intestine with Qi and blood stagnation manifested as dysentery, diarrhea, abdominal pain with tenesmus, a burning sensation in the anus, blood and pus in the stools, dark and scanty urine, red tongue with yellow greasy coat, a slippery, rapid pulse.

■ Cautions and Contraindications
It should not be used in cases of early stage of dysentery with exterior symptoms or chronic dysentery due to deficient cold.

■ Modern Applications
Acute dysentery, acute enteritis, amebic dysentery, ulcerative colitis, etc.

She Chuang Zi San-Cnidium Seed Powder
Cnidium Formula
蛇床子散

■ Ingredients

She Chuang Zi	Cnidium Seed	10-15g
Hua Jiao	Zanthoxylum	10-15g
Ming Fan	Alumen	10-15g
Ku Shen	Bitter Ginseng Root	10-15g
Bai Bu	Stemona Root	10-15g

■ Preparation
External use only. Decocts all ingredients, use as an herbal steam bath first, then followed by an immersion bath once a day, ten days per therapeutic course.

■ Pertaining Category
Additional Formulas for Ob-Gyn Disorders

■ Functions
Dries dampness, kills parasites, alleviates itching.

■ Indications

Toxic damp-heat in the lower burner manifested as constant vaginal itching and agitation, or even pain in the severe case, excessive yellow, fishy-smelling, or foamy vaginal discharge, irritability, insomnia, a bitter taste in the mouth with sticky feeling, a fullness and discomfort sensation in the chest, reduced appetite, red tongue with yellow greasy coat, a wiry, rapid pulse.

■ Cautions and Contraindications

Do not use Hua Jiao (Zanthoxylum) for vaginal itching with ulceration in the genital area.

■ Modern Applications

Trichomonas vaginitis, etc.

She Gan Ma Huang Tang-Belamcanda and Ephedra Decoction
Belamcanda and Ephedra Combination
射干麻黄汤

■ Ingredients

She Gan	Belamcanda	9g
Ma Huang	Ephedra	9g
Xi Xin	Asarum	3g
Zi Wan	Purple Aster Root	9g
Kuan Dong Hua	Coltsfoot Flower	9g
Ban Xia	Pinellia Tuber	9g
Wu Wei Zi	Schisandra	3g
Sheng Jiang	Fresh Ginger	9g
Da Zao	Jujube	3pcs

■ Preparation

Use as decoction or prepared form.

■ **Pertaining Category**
Pungent Warm Exterior Relieving

■ **Functions**
Opens and warms the lungs, transforms phlegm-fluid, directs
rebellious Qi downward, stops coughing and wheezing. Releases the
exterior wind-cold.

■ **Indications**
Pronounced interior phlegm-fluid retention with or without mild
exterior condition manifested as severe coughing and wheezing with
rattling sound in the throat, or aversion to cold, white thick and
greasy tongue coat, a superficial, tight pulse.

■ **Cautions and Contraindications**
It is contraindicated in cases of coughing of blood, dry cough with
dry mouth and throat, and cough with thick yellow sputum. Do not
use overdose and for long-term. Use with caution for patients with
hypertension and heart problems.

■ **Modern Applications**
Influenza, acute and chronic bronchitis, bronchial asthma,
pulmonary emphysema, etc.

Shen Fu Tang-Ginseng and Aconite
Decoction
Ginseng and Aconite Combination
参 附 汤

■ **Ingredients**

Ren Shen	*Ginseng*	9-12g
Pao Fu Zi	*Prepared Aconite*	6-9g

■ **Preparation**
Use as decoction.

■ **Pertaining Category**
Rescuing Collapsed Yang

■ **Functions**
Restores the collapsed Yang, tonifies Qi, rescues the patient from shork.

■ **Indications**
Sudden collapse of Qi and Yang manifested as cold hands and feet, intolerance to cold, dizziness, shortness and weak breath, pale complexion, spontaneous sweating, pale tongue with thin white coat, a thin, faint pulse.

■ **Cautions and Contraindications**
It is contraindicated in cases of cold limbs due to interior accumulation of heat. For patients with flushed face due to true cold and false heat, the formula should be taken in cool.

■ **Modern Applications**
Shock due to heart failure or cardiac infarction. etc.
In this formula, Ren Shen (Ginseng) can not be replaced by Dang Shen (Codonopsis) or Xi Yang Shen (American Ginseng). This formula is focus on restoring Qi; while Si Ni Jia Ren Shen Tang is focus on rescuing Yang.

Shen Ling Bai Zhu San-Ginseng, Hoelen, and White Atractylodes Powder
Ginseng and Atractylodes Formula
参 苓 白 术 散

■ Ingredients

Ren Shen	Ginseng	1000g
Fu Ling	Hoelen/Poria	1000g
Bai Zhu	White Atractylodes	1000g
Yi Yi Ren	Coix	500g
Sha Ren	Amomum Fruit	500g
Jie Geng	Platycodon	500g
Lian Zi	Lotus Seed	500g
Bian Dou	Dolichos	750g
Shan Yao	Dioscorea	1000g
Zhi Gan Cao	Baked Licorice	1000g

■ Preparation
Use as prepared form or decoction with properly reduced dosage, usually one-hundredth the dosage as above.

■ Pertaining Category
Qi Tonifying

■ Functions
Tonifies the spleen Qi, harmonizes the stomach. Eliminates dampness, stops diarrhea.

■ Indications
Spleen Qi deficiency with severe dampness retention manifested as poor appetite, loose stools, diarrhea, vomiting, lassitude, emaciation, fullness in the chest and epigastrium, abdominal distention, sallow complexion, pale tongue with white coat, a thin, weak, and soft pulse.

■ Cautions and Contraindications
Use with caution in cases of Qi and Yin deficiency.

■ Modern Applications
Indigestion, children's malnutrition, chronic gastroenteritis, anemia, nephritic syndrome, chronic hepatitis, chronic bronchitis, diabetes mellitus, etc.

Shen Su Yin-Ginseng and Perilla Leaf Beverage
Ginseng and Perilla Combination
参苏饮

■ **Ingredients**

Ren Shen	Ginseng	3g
Zi Su Ye	Perilla Leaf	6g
Ge Gen	Pueraria	6g
Qian Hu	Hogfennel Root	6g
Ban Xia	Pinellia Tuber	6g
Fu Ling	Hoelen/Poria	6g
Chen Pi	Tangerine Peel	3g
Jie Geng	Platycodon	6g
Zhi Ke	Bitter Orange	6g
Mu Xiang	Saussurea	3g
Gan Cao	Licorice	3g
Sheng Jiang	Fresh Ginger	3 slices
Da Zao	Jujube	3pcs

■ **Preparation**

Use as decoction or prepared form.

■ **Pertaining Category**

Strengthening Body Resistance and Relieving Exterior

■ **Functions**

Tonifies Qi, expels wind-cold, releases the exterior. Resolves phlegm, stops coughing. Harmonizes the stomach.

■ **Indications**

Invasion of wind-cold with Qi deficiency constitution and phlegm-dampness retention manifested as aversion to cold, fever, headache, stuffy nose, cough with profuse sputum, fullness in the chest, pale tongue with white coat, a superficial, weak pulse.

Cautions and Contraindications
Do not use this formula for patients with strong constitution.

Modern Applications
Common cold, acute or chronic bronchitis, etc.

Shen Tong Zhu Yu Tang-Remove Blood Stasis from Aching Muscle Decoction
Drive Out Blood Stasis from a Painful Body Decoction
身痛逐瘀汤

Ingredients

Qin Jiao	*Big Leaf Gentiana*	3g
Chuan Xiong	*Ligusticum*	6g
Tao Ren	*Peach Kernel*	9g
Hong Hua	*Safflower*	9g
Qiang Huo	*Notopterygium*	3g
Mo Yao	*Myrrh*	6g
Dang Gui	*Chinese Angelica*	9g
Wu Ling Zhi	*Trogopterus*	6g
Xiang Fu	*Cyperus*	3g
Chuan Niu Xi	*Cyathula*	9g
Di Long	*Earthworm*	6g
Gan Cao	*Licorice*	6g

Preparation
Use as decoction or prepared form. Wu Ling Zhi should be wrapped in gauze when making decoction.

Pertaining Category
Blood Invigorating

Functions
Promotes circulation of blood and Qi, removes blood stasis.
Unblocks the channels, stops pain, relieves arthralgia.

289

■ Indications

Stagnation of blood and Qi in the channels and collaterals manifested as prolonged aching muscles or painful joints in the shoulder, limbs, lower back, or whole body, purple tongue, a wiry, hesitant pulse.

■ Cautions and Contraindications

It is contraindicated during pregnancy and in cases of excessive menstrual bleeding, bleeding diathesis, or any bleeding disorders, etc.

■ Modern Applications

Rheumatic arthritis, traumatoid arthritis, lumbago, etc.

Sheng Hua Tang-Generating and Transforming Decoction
Tang-kuei and Ginger Combination
生化汤

■ Ingredients

Dang Gui	Chinese Angelica	24g
Chuan Xiong	Ligusticum	9g
Tao Ren	Peach Kernel	6-9g
Pao Gan Jiang	Blast-fried Ginger	2g
Zhi Gan Cao	Baked Licorice	2g

■ Preparation

Use as decoction or add some yellow rice wine.

■ Pertaining Category

Blood Invigorating

■ Functions

Promotes blood circulation, removes blood stasis. Warms the channels, stops pain.

■ Indications

Postpartum blood deficiency with blood stagnation due to cold invasion manifested as retention of lochia or scanty lochia, accompanied by coldness and pain in the lower abdomen, aggravated by pressure, or mass in the lower abdomen, dark purple tongue, a deep, hesitant pulse.

■ Cautions and Contraindications

It is contraindicated during pregnancy or in cases of blood stasis with heat, and any other bleeding disorders.

■ Modern Applications

Lochiostasis, retention of placenta, uterus fibroids, postpartum abdominal pain due to uterine contraction, chronic endometriosis, etc.

Sheng Jiang Xie Xin Tang-Fresh Ginger Decoction to Purge the Stomach
Pinellia and Ginger Combination
生姜泻心汤

■ Ingredients

Ban Xia	Pinellia Tuber	9g
Huang Qin	Scute	6g
Gan Jiang	Dried Ginger	2g
Ren Shen	Ginseng	6g
Huang Lian	Coptis	3g
Zhi Gan Cao	Baked Licorice	6g
Da Zao	Jujube	4pcs
Sheng Jiang	Fresh Ginger	12g

■ Preparation

Use as decoction or prepared form.

■ **Pertaining Category**
Regulating the Intestines and Stomach (Mediating).

■ **Functions**
Harmonizes the stomach, descends the rebellious stomach Qi downward. Relieves focal distention. Expels water accumulation.

■ **Indications**
Disharmony between stomach and intestines with water and heat accumulation manifested as fullness and hardness in the epigastrium, retching with foul smelling, severe borborygmus, diarrhea, red tongue with yellow greasy coat, a slippery, rapid pulse.

■ **Cautions and Contraindications**
It is contraindicated in cases of retching and nausea due to stomach Yin deficiency.

■ **Modern Applications**
Acute or chronic gastroenteritis, peptic ulcer, indigestion, gastrointestinal neurosis, morning sickness, etc.
This formula is modified from Ban Xia Xie Xin Tang (Pinellia Decoction to Purge the Stomach).

Sheng Ma Ge Gen Tang-Cimicifuga and Pueraria Decoction
Cimicifuga and Pueraria Combination
升麻葛根汤

■ **Ingredients**

Sheng Ma	Cimicifuga	3g
Ge Gen	Pueraria Root	3g
Chi Shao Yao	Red Peony	6g
Zhi Gan Cao	Baked Licorice	3g

■ Preparation
Use as decoction or prepared form.

■ Pertaining Category
Pungent Cool Exterior Relieving

■ Functions
Expels wind-heat, releases the pathogen from muscle layer, promotes the eruption of measles.

■ Indications
Early stage of measles or rashes that do not erupt evenly, fever, headache, body aches, aversion to wind, sneezing, or slight cough, thirst, or red eyes, red and dry tongue with dry coat, a superficial, rapid pulse.

■ Cautions and Contraindications
It is contraindicated in cases of measles that erupt evenly or sink internally with shortness of breath, coughing and wheezing.

■ Modern Applications
Influenza, measles, scarlet fever, initial stage of chicken pox, and acute enteritis, etc.

Sheng Mai San-Activate the Pulse Powder
Ginseng and Ophiopogon Formula
生脉散

■ Ingredients

Ren Shen	Ginseng	10g
Mai Men Dong	Ophiopogon	15g
Wu Wei Zi	Schisandra	6g

■ Preparation
Use as decoction or prepared form.

- **■ Pertaining Category**

Qi Tonifying

- **■ Functions**

Tonifies Qi, generates body fluids. Astringes Yin, stops sweating.

- **■ Indications**

Qi and Yin deficiency (especially in the heart and lungs) manifested as fatigue, shortness of breath, dislike to speak, profuse sweating, thirst, dry mouth and throat, chronic dry cough, palpitation, red and dry tongue with scanty coat, a weak, feeble pulse.

- **■ Cautions and Contraindications**

It is contraindicated in cases of exterior patterns, acute cough, or summer heat without damage of Qi and Yin fluids.

- **■ Modern Applications**

Dehydrant shock due to heat stroke, bleeding, severe vomiting and diarrhea, traumatic injury, and scald; later stage of febrile disease, recovery from chronic diseases or after surgery; pulmonary tuberculosis, chronic bronchitis, bronchiectasis, coronary heart disease, angina pectoris, arrhythmia, etc.

Sheng Tie Luo Yin-Iron Filings Beverage
Iron Filings Combination
生 铁 落 饮

■ Ingredients

Sheng Tie Luo	Frusta Ferri	30-60g
Dan Nan Xing	Arisaema Tuber	3g
Zhe Bei Mu	Thunberg Fritillary	9g
Mai Men Dong	Ophiopogon	9g
Tian Men Dong	Asparagus	9g
Xuan Shen	Scrophularia	5g
Gou Teng	Uncaria	5g
Fu Ling	Hoelen/Poria	3g
Fu Shen	Hoelen/Poria	3g
Lian Qiao	Forsythia Fruit	3g
Shi Chang Pu	Sweetflag Rhizome	3g
Dan Shen	Salvia	5g
Chen Pi	Tangerine Peel	3g
Yuan Zhi	Polygala	3g
Zhu Sha	Cinnabar	1g

■ Preparation
Use as decoction or prepared form. Sheng Tie Luo should be decocted first for about 1.5 hour, then add other ingredients.

■ Pertaining Category
Spirit Calming with Heavy Sedative Herbs

■ Functions
Sedates the heart, calms spirit. Clears fire-heat, resolves phlegm. Subdues the liver Yang.

■ Indications
Phlegm-fire disturbing the heart and spirit manifested as mania, agitation, laughing or screaming without apparent reason, or violent behavior, severe headache, easy to get angry, insomnia, red tongue with yellow greasy coat, a slippery, wiry, and rapid pulse.

■ Cautions and Contraindications

Do not use overdose and for long term to prevent mercurialism from Zhu Sha (Cinnabar). It is contraindicated during pregnancy.

■ Modern Applications

Mania, psychosis, schizophrenia, etc.

Sheng Xian Tang-Raise the Sinking Decoction
Astragalus and Cimicifuga Combination
升 陷 汤

■ Ingredients

Huang Qi	Astragalus	18g
Zhi Mu	Anemarrhena	9g
Chai Hu	Bupleurum	4.5g
Jie Geng	Platycodon	4.5g
Sheng Ma	Cimicifuga	3g

■ Preparation

Use as decoction or prepared form.

■ Pertaining Category

Qi Tonifying

■ Functions

Tonigies and lifts the Qi.

■ Indications

Lung and spleen Qi deficiency and sinking manifested as rapid and difficult breathing, shortness of breath, pale complexion, poor appetite, low voice, or loose stools, pale tongue with thin white coat, a deep, slow, and weak pulse.

- **Cautions and Contraindications**

None noted.

- **Modern Applications**

Chronic bronchitis, chronic bronchial asthma, pulmonary emphysema, gastric prolapse, chronic diarrhea, or functional uterine bleeding, etc.

Sheng Yu Tang-Sage-like Healing Decoction
Ginseng and Rehmannia Formula
圣 愈 汤

- **Ingredients**

Shu Di Huang	Cooked Rehmannia	20g
Bai Shao Yao	White Peony	15g
Dang Gui	Chinese Angelica	15g
Chuan Xiong	Ligusticum	8g
Ren Shen	Ginseng	10g
Huang Qi	Astragalus	18g

- **Preparation**

Use as decoction or prepared form.

- **Pertaining Category**

Qi and Blood Tonifying

- **Functions**

Nourishes blood, tonifies Qi, controls and preserves blood, calms fetus.

■ **Indications**
Blood and spleen Qi deficiency with inability to control blood manifested as dizziness, fatigue, listlessness, lusterless complexion scanty, pale menstruation, or shortened menstrual cycle with excessive flow, but pale color and thin quality, lower abdominal pain during or after menstruation, or during pregnancy, which is alleviated by pressure, pale tongue with thin white coat, a thin, weak, and faint pulse.

■ **Cautions and Contraindications**
None noted.

■ **Modern Applications**
Anemia, amenorrhea, dysmenorrhea, uterine bleeding, threatened abortion, habitual abortion, etc.

Shi Hu Ye Guang Wan-Treat Night Vision Pill with Dendrobium
Dendrobium and Rehmannia Combination
石 斛 夜 光 丸

■ Ingredients

Shi Hu	Dendrobium	15g
Tian Men Dong	Asparagus	60g
Mai Men Dong	Ophiopogon	30g
Shu Di Huang	Cooked Rehmannia	30g
Sheng Di Huang	Dried Rehmannia	30g
Ren Shen	Ginseng	60g
Fu Ling	Hoelen/Poria	60g
Tu Si Zi	Dodder Seed	30g
Jue Ming Zi	Cassia Seed	24g
Gou Qi Zi	Lycium Fruit	24g
Wu Wei Zi	Schisandra	24g
Xing Ren	Apricot Seed	24g
Shan Yao	Dioscorea	24g
Bai Ji Li	Tribulus	15g
Rou Cong Rong	Cistanche	15g
Chuan Xiong	Ligusticum	15g
Zhi Ke	Bitter Orange	15g
Qing Xiang Zi	Celosia	15g
Fang Feng	Siler	15g
Huang Lian	Coptis	15g
Xi Jiao	Rhinoceros Horn	15g
Ling Yang Jiao	Antelope Horn	15g
Zhi Gan Cao	Baked Licorice	15g
Niu Xi	Achyranthes Root	24g
Ju Hua	Chrysanthemum	24g

■ Preparation
Use as prepared form.

■ Pertaining Category
Yin Tonifying

■ Functions
Nourishes the liver and kidney Yin, brightens the eyes. Calms liver Yang, extinguishes liver wind.

■ **Indications**

Yin deficiency of the liver and kidney with deficient fire and eye disturbance manifested as dizziness, blurred vision, aversion to light, excessive tearing, poor night vision, early stage of cataract, or blood-shot eyes, red and thin tongue with scanty coat or cracked tongue, a thin, rapid pulse.

■ **Cautions and Contraindications**

It is contraindicated in cases of exterior patterns.

■ **Modern Applications**

Diminished vision, night blandness, glaucoma, cataract, diabetes, myopia, etc.

Shi Hui San-Ten Charred Ingredients Powder
Thistle Formula
十 灰 散

■ **Ingredients**

Da Ji	Japanese Thistle	10g
Xiao Ji	Small Thistle	10g
He Ye	Lotus Leaf	10g
Ce Bai Ye	Biota Leaves	10g
Bai Mao Gen	Imperata	10g
Qian Cao Gen	Madder Root	10g
Zhi Zi	Gardenia Fruit	10g
Da Huang	Rhubarb	10g
Mu Dan Pi	Moutan Bark	10g
Zong Lu Pi	Trachycarpus	10g

■ **Preparation**

All ingredients are charred. Use as prepared form or decoction.

■ **Pertaining Category**

Stopping Bleeding

■ Functions

Cools blood, stops bleeding.

■ Indications

Excessive fire-heat in the blood manifested as all kinds of acute bleeding such as vomiting of blood, coughing of blood, nosebleeding, dry mouth and throat, dark red tongue with yellow coat, a wiry, rapid, and forceful pulse.

■ Cautions and Contraindications

It is contraindicated in cases of bleeding due to deficient cold.

■ Modern Applications

Epistaxis, hematemesis, hemoptysis, peptic ulcer, bronchiectasis, etc.

Discontinue the formula when bleeding stopped.

Shi Pi San (Yin)-Bolster the Spleen Powder (Beverage)
Magnolia and Atractylodes Combination
实 脾 散 (饮)

■ Ingredients

Hou Po	Magnolia Bark	6g
Bai Zhu	White Atractylodes	6g
Mu Gua	Chaenomeles Fruit	6g
Mu Xiang	Saussurea	6g
Cao Guo	Tsaoko Fruit	6g
Da Fu Pi	Areca Peel	6g
Fu Zi	Prepared Aconite	6g
Fu Ling	Hoelen/Poria	6g
Gan Jiang	Dried Ginger	6g
Zhi Gan Cao	Baked Licirice	3g
Sheng Jiang	Fresh Ginger	5slices
Da Zao	Jujube	1pc

■ **Preparation**
Use as decoction or prepared form.

■ **Pertaining Category**
Yang Warming and Dampness Transforming

■ **Functions**
Warms Yang, tonifies the spleen. Moves Qi, promotes urination.

■ **Indications**
Spleen and kidney Yang deficiency with water retention and Qi stagnation manifested as generalized edema mostly below the waist, cold extremities, aversion to cold, absence of thirst, a fullness sensation in the chest, abdominal distention, poor appetite, decreased urination, heaviness of the body, loose stools, pale tongue with thick greasy coat, a deep, slow, and weak pulse.

■ **Cautions and Contraindications**
None noted.

■ **Modern Applications**
Ascites from liver cirrhosis, chronic hepatic disorders, cardiac edema chronic nephritis, chronic enteritis, intestinal tuberculosis, etc.

Shi Quan Da Bu Tang-Great Tonifying Decoction with Ten Ingredients
Ginseng and Tang-kuei Ten Combination
十 全 大 补 汤

■ Ingredients

Ren Shen	Ginseng	8g
Bai Zhu	White Atractylodes	10g
Fu Ling	Hoelen/Poria	8g
Shu Di Huang	Cooked Rehmannia	15g
Dang Gui	Chinese Angelica	10g
Bai Shao Yao	White Peony	8g
Chuan Xiong	Ligusticum	5g
Huang Qi	Astragalus	15g
Rou Gui	Cinnamon Bark	8g
Zhi Gan Cao	Baked Licorice	5g
Sheng Jiang	Fresh Ginger	3slices
Da Zao	Jujube	2pcs

■ Preparation
Use as decoction or prepared form.

■ Pertaining Category
Qi and Blood Tonifying

■ Functions
Tonifies Qi, nourishes blood, warms Yang.

■ Indications
Deficiency of Qi and blood with mild deficient cold manifested as pale or sallow complexion, dizziness, blurred vision, fatigue, shortness of breath, palpitation, loss of appetite, cold hands and feet, weak limbs, or chronic consumptive cough, or prolonged non-healing sores, or uterine bleeding, or seminal emission, pale tongue with thin white coat, a thin, weak pulse.

■ Cautions and Contraindications
None noted.

■ Modern Applications
Anemia, cardiac failure, chronic abscess, postpartum weakness, uterine bleeding, amenorrhea, pulmonary tuberculosis, neurasthenia, etc.

Shi Wei San-Pyrrosia Leaf Powder

Pyrrosia Combination

石苇散

■ **Ingredients**

Shi Wei	*Pyrrosia Leaf*	9g
Qu Mai	*Dianthus*	9g
Che Qian Zi	*Plantago Seed*	12g
Dong Kui Zi	*Musk Mallow Seed*	9g
Hua Shi	*Talcum`*	15g

■ **Preparation**

Use as decoction or prepared form. Che Qian Zi should be wrapped in gauze when making decoction.

■ **Pertaining Category**

Damp-heat Clearing

■ **Functions**

Clears heat, promotes urination, drains damp-heat, expels stones.

■ **Indications**

Bladder damp-heat with stones manifested as passage urinary calculi or gravel, difficult urination, periodic lower back cramping pain extending to lower abdomen, pubic region, and thigh, bloody urine, or fever, red tongue with yellow greasy coat, a wiry, slippery and rapid pulse.

■ **Cautions and Contraindications**

Use cautiously for patients with deficiency of the spleen and stomach.

■ **Modern Applications**

Urinary tract calculi, cystitis, urethritis, prostatitis, etc.

Shi Xiao San-Lose the Smile Powder
Pteropus and Bulrush Formula
失 笑 散

- **Ingredients**

| Wu Ling Zhi | *Trogopterus* | 10-15g |
| Pu Huang | *Bulrush Pollen* | 10-15g |

- **Preparation**

Use as prepared form or decoction. Wu Ling Zhi should be wrapped in gauze when making decoction.

- **Pertaining Category**

Blood Invigorating

- **Functions**

Promotes blood circulation, removes blood stasis. Disperses lumps or hardening, stops pain.

- **Indications**

Stagnation of blood manifested as severe pain in the chest, epigastrium, and abdomen, retention of lochia, postpartum abdominal pain, or irregular menstruation with colicky pain in the lower abdomen, dark red tongue with purple spots, a wiry, tight, and hesitant pulse.

- **Cautions and Contraindications**

It is contraindicated during pregnancy. Use with caution for patients with weakness in the spleen and stomach.

- **Modern Applications**

Dysmenorrhea, amenorrhea, endometriosis, lochioschesis, coronary artery disease, postpartum abdominal pain, etc.

Shi Zao Tang-Ten Jujubes Decoction
Jujube Combination
十枣汤

■ **Ingredients**

Gan Sui	*Kansui Root*	Equal
Yuan Hua	*Daphne Flower*	dosage
Da Ji	*Euphorbia*	
Da Zao	*Jujube*	10pcs

■ **Preparation**

Grind first three ingredients into fine powder, mix and put into capsules, take 0.5-1g each time with the decoction of 10 jujubes, once a day in the morning on an empty stomach.

■ **Pertaining Category**

Purging Downward with Harsh Cathartics

■ **Functions**

Drastically eliminates the interior excessive water retention.

■ **Indications**

Sereve interior water retention with strong constitution manifested as pain in the chest and hypochondrium when coughing or spitting, hardness in the epigastrium, retching, shortness of breath, headache with dizziness, difficulty in breathing due to pain in the thorax and back, or severe general edema, worse in the lower part of the body, abdominal distention, difficulty in urination and defecation, white moist tongue coat, a deep, wiry pulse.

■ **Cautions and Contraindications**
It is contraindicated for patients with weak constitution or during pregnancy. If severe diarrhea occurs, the cold rice porridge should be taken to benefit recovery.

■ **Modern Applications**
Pleural effusion, uremia from systemic lupus erythematosus, nephritic syndrome, ascites from liver cirrhosis, or late stage of schistosomiasis, etc.
In cases complicated with excess and deficiency, this formula should be taken with or alternated with another tonifying formula together.

Shou Tai Wan-Fetus Longevity Pill
Loranthus and Cuscuta Combination
寿 胎 丸

■ **Ingredients**

Sang Ji Sheng	Loranthus	12g
Tu Si Zi	Dodder Seed	12g
Xu Duan	Teasel Root	12g
E Jiao	Equus/Gelatin	9g

■ **Preparation**
Use as decoction or prepared form. E Jiao should be dissolved separately in boiling water and added into the strained decoction.

■ **Pertaining Category**
Additional Formulas for Ob-Gyn Disorders

■ **Functions**
Tonifies and stabilizes the kidneys, calms the fetus.

■ Indications

Threatened miscarriage due to kidney Qi deficiency manifested as slight vaginal bleeding during pregnancy, pale or dark color, lower back or abdominal pain with a bearing down sensation, dizziness, tinnitus, frequent urination, especially at night, or even urinary incontinence, or with history of miscarriage, pale tongue with white coat, a deep, weak pulse.

■ Cautions and Contraindications

None noted.

■ Modern Applications

Threatened miscarriage, habitual abortion, lower back pain, etc.
For best results, Dang Shen(Codonopsis)9g and Bai Zhu(White Atractylodes)9g should be added.

Shu Zuo Yin Zi-Coursing and Piercing Beverage
Alisma and Areca Combination
疏凿饮子

■ Ingredients

Ze Xie	Alisma	12g
Da Fu Pi	Areca Peel	15g
Chi Xiao Dou	Phaseolus	15g
Shang Lu	Phytolacca	6g
Qiang Huo	Notopterygium	9g
Chuan Jiao	Zanthoxylum	9g
Mu Tong	Akebia	12g
Qin Jiao	Big Leaf Gentiana	9g
Bing Lang	Betel (Areca) Nut	9g
Fu Ling Pi	Poria Peel	30g
Sheng Jiang	Fresh Ginger	3g

■ **Preparation**
Use as decoction or prepared form.

■ **Pertaining Category**
Purging Downward with Harsh Cathartics

■ **Functions**
Eliminates internal damp-heat by promoting diuresis and bowel movement. Disperses superficial swelling by expelling wind and relieving the exterior.

■ **Indications**
Excessive water retention affecting both exterior and interior with strong constitution manifested as severe general edema with moist shiny skin, fullness in the chest and abdomen, difficulty in breathing, thirst, dark and scanty urine, constipation, yellow greasy tongue coat, a soft, rapid pulse.

■ **Cautions and Contraindications**
It is contraindicated during pregnancy. Do not use overdose and for long term.

■ **Modern Applications**
Edema, ascites from liver cirrhosis, edema from acute nephritis, uremia, etc.
This formula is slightly toxic.

Shui Lu Er Xian Dan-Water and Land Two Immortals Elixir
Euryale Seed Formula
水陆二仙丹

■ **Ingredients**

| Qian Shi | Euryale Seed | 10g |
| Jin Ying Zi | Cherokee Rosehip | 10g |

■ **Preparation**
Use as decoction or prepared form.

■ **Pertaining Category**
Binding the Essence to Stop Seminal Emission and Enuresis

■ **Functions**
Stabilizes the kidneys, binds up essence.

■ **Indications**
Insufficiency of the kidney essence and Yang manifested as cloudy spermatorrhea, leukorrhea, soreness and weakness of lower back and knees, tinnitus, fatigue, pale tongue, a frail pulse.

■ **Cautions and Contraindications**
It is contraindicated for excess patterns of seminal emission or leukorrhea.

■ **Modern Applications**
Seminal emission, sexual dysfunction, etc.

Si Jun Zi Tang-Four Gentleman Decoction
Four Major Herb Combination
四君子汤

■ **Ingredients**

Ren Shen	Ginseng	9g
Bai Zhu	White Atractylodes	9g
Fu Ling	Hoelen/Poria	9g
Zhi Gan Cao	Baked Licorice	6g

■ **Preparation**
Use as decoction or prepared form.

■ **Pertaining Category**
Qi Tonifying

310

■ **Functions**
Tonifies Qi, strengthens the spleen and stomach.

■ **Indications**
Spleen and stomach Qi deficiency manifested as pale complexion, weak voice, lassitude, poor appetite, abdominal bloating after eating, loose stools, pale tongue with thin white coat, a thin, weak, and deep pulse.

■ **Cautions and Contraindications**
It is contraindicated in cases of high fever, empty fire, bloating due to food stagnation, lack of body fluid, excessive thirst, constipation. Long term use may cause thirst, dryness of tongue or mouth, and irritability.

■ **Modern Applications**
Chronic gastroenteritis, chronic dysentery, peptic ulcer, anemia, hypoproteinemia, malnutrition, etc.

Si Miao Wan(San)-Four Mysterious Pill(Powder)
Four Marvel Pill(Powder)
四 妙 丸 (散)

■ **Ingredients**

Huang Bai	Phellodendron	240g
Yi Yi Ren	Coix	240g
Cang Zhu	Atractylodes	120g
Huai Niu Xi	Achyranthes Root	120g

■ **Preparation**
Use as prepared form or decoction with properly reduced dosage.

■ **Pertaining Category**
Damp-heat Clearing

■ Functions

Clears heat, drains dampness. Invigorates blood circulation, strengthens bones and tendons.

■ Indications

Damp-heat in the lower burner manifested as soreness and weakness of lower back, painful, red, hot, and swollen knees and feet, weakness, numbness, or atrophy of lower limbs, dark yellow, scanty, and difficult urine, foul-smelling vaginal discharge, red tongue with yellow greasy coat, a slippery, rapid pulse.

■ Cautions and Contraindications

None noted.

■ Modern Applications

Acute or chronic UTI, vaginitis, cervicitis, rheumatic, rheumatoid, or gouty arthritis, beriberi, etc.

Si Miao Yong An Tang-Four Mysterious Ingredients Decoction for Calming Hero
Four Valiant Decoction for Well-being
四妙勇安汤

■ Ingredients

Jin Yin Hua	Lonicera	90g
Xuan Shen	Scrophularia	90g·
Dang Gui	Chinese Angelica	30-60g
Gan Cao	Licorice	15-30g

■ Preparation

Use as prepared form or decoction with properly adjusted dosage.

■ Pertaining Category

Treating External Carbuncles

■ Functions

Clears heat, relieves toxicity. Promotes the blood circulation, reduces swelling, stops pain.

■ Indications

Gangrene due to toxic-heat and blood stagnation manifested as swelling and severe burning pain of affected extremities with dark redness and foul smelling ulceration, fever, thirst, red tongue with yellow greasy coat, a rapid, wiry pulse.

■ Cautions and Contraindications

It is contraindicated for gangrene of Yin cold type and patients with deficiency of Qi and blood.

■ Modern Applications

Thromboangiitis obliterans, thrombosis in the lower limbs, gangrene, other diseases due to vascular occlusion, etc.

Si Mo Tang(Yin)-Four Milled Herb Decoction(Beverage)
Ginseng and Betel Nut Combination
四 磨 汤(饮)

■ Ingredients

Ren Shen	Ginseng	3g
Bing Lang	Betel Nut	9g
Chen Xiang	Aquilaria	3g
Wu Yao	Lindera	9g

■ Preparation

Use as decoction or prepared form.

■ Pertaining Category

Qi Regulating(Descending)

■ Functions
Moves and descends the adverse flow of Qi. Opens chest, disperses clumps. Tonifies Qi.

■ Indications
Stagnant liver Qi counteracting on the lungs and overacting on the stomach manifested as a stifling sensation in the chest and diaphragm, wheezing, shortness of breath, irritability, epigastric fullness, loss of appetite, light purple tongue with thin white coat, a wiry pulse.

■ Cautions and Contraindications
None noted.

■ Modern Applications
Bronchial asthma, gastritis, intestinal dysfunction, indigestion, neurosis, etc.

Si Ni Jia Ren Shen Tang-Four Frigid Limbs Decoction with Ginseng
G.L. and Aconite Combination with Ginseng
四逆加人参汤

■ Ingredients

Fu Zi	Aconite	6-9g
Gan Jiang	Dried Ginger	4.5g
Zhi Gan Cao	Baked Licorice	6g
Ren Shen	Ginseng	6-9g

■ Preparation
Decoct Ginseng separately for at least one hour, then mixed with decoction of Si Ni Tang (prepared as instructed).

■ Pertaining Category
Rescuing Collapsed Yang

■ Functions
Restores Yang, tonifies Qi, rescues the collapsed Yang, Qi, and Yin.

■ Indications
Yang and Qi collapse with severe blood loss or dehydration
manifested as extreme cold hands and feet, intolerance to cold,
watery diarrhea has stopped, fatigue, lethargy, pale tongue, a thin, or
hollow pulse.

■ Cautions and Contraindications
It is contraindicated in cases of cold limbs due to interior
accumulation of heat. For patient with flushed face due to true cold
and false heat, the formula should be taken in cool.

■ Modern Applications
Chronic consumptive disease, hypopituitarism, hypothyroidism,
hypoadrenocorticism, shock due to heart failure or cardiac infarction
chronic gastroenteritis, cholera, gastroptosis, chronic dysentery,
blood loss, dehydration, etc.
*This formula is modified from Si Ni Tang (Four Frigid Limbs
Decoction).*

Si Ni San-Powder for Treating Cold Limbs
Bupleurum and Chih-shih Formula
四 逆 散

■ Ingredients

Chai Hu	Bupleurum	6g
Zhi Shi	Immature Citrus	6g
Bai Shao Yao	White Peony	9g
Zhi Gan Cao	Baked Licorice	6g

■ Preparation
Use as decoction or prepared form.

■ **Pertaining Category**
Regulating the Liver and Spleen (Mediating)

■ **Functions**
Disperses pathogens. Soothes liver Qi, relieves stagnation, regulates spleen.

■ **Indications**
Internal stagnated Yang Qi which fails to reach the extremities causing cold limbs, or disharmony between the liver and stomach manifested as a fullness sensation in the hypochondrium and epigastrium, abdominal distention or pain, diarrhea with tenesmus, white tongue coat, a wiry pulse.

■ **Cautions and Contraindications**
It is contraindicated for patients with cold limbs caused by excess cold or Yang deficiency.

■ **Modern Applications**
Syncope due to heat, gastritis, peptic ulcer, hepatitis, cholecystitis, cholelithiasis, pancreatitis, mastitis, fibrocystic breasts, intercostal neuralgia, etc.

Si Ni Tang-Four Frigid Limbs Decoction
Aconite, Ginger, and Licorice Combination
四 逆 汤

■ **Ingredients**

Sheng Fu Zi	Aconite	6-9g
Gan Jiang	Dried Ginger	4.5g
Zhi Gan Cao	Zhi Gan Cao	6g

■ **Preparation**
Use as decoction. Sheng Fu Zi(Unprepared Aconite) may be substituted by Zhi Fu Zi (Prepared Aconite). Fu Zi should be decocted 30-60 minutes before adding other ingredients.

■ **Pertaining Category**
Rescuing Collapsed Yang

■ **Functions**
Restores the collapsed Yang, rescues the patient from shock. Warms the spleen and kidney Yang.

■ **Indications**
Severe Yang deficiency of the kidney and spleen or Yang collapse manifested as extreme cold hands and feet, intolerance of cold, fatigue, lethargy, like to curled up, absence of thirst, vomiting, abdominal pain, watery diarrhea, tastelessness in the mouth, pale tongue with white moist coat, a deep, faint, and thin pulse.

■ **Cautions and Contraindications**
It is contraindicated in cases of cold limbs due to interior accumulation of heat. For patient with flushed face due to true cold and false heat, the formula should be taken in cool.

■ **Modern Applications**
Chronic consumptive disease, hypopituitarism, hypothyroidism, hypoadrenocorticism, shock due to heart failure or cardiac infarction, chronic gastroenteritis, cholera, gastroptosis, chronic dysentery, etc.

Si Shen Wan-Four Miracle Pill
Psoralea and Myristica Formula
四神丸

■ **Ingredients**

Rou Dou Kou	Nutmeg	60g
Bu Gu Zhi	Psoralea	120g
Wu Wei Zi	Schisandra	60g
Wu Zhu Yu	Evodia	30g

■ **Preparation**
Use as prepared form or decoction with properly reduced dosage.

■ **Pertaining Category**
Astringing the Intestines to Stop Diarrhea

■ **Functions**
Warms the spleen and kidney, astringes the intestines, stops diarrhea.

■ **Indications**
Deficient coldness in the spleen and kidney manifested as diarrhea before dawn, or prolonged diarrhea with undigested food, abdominal pain, lumbago, cold limbs, poor appetite, listlessness, lassitude, pale tongue with thin white coat, a deep, weak, and slow pulse.

■ **Cautions and Contraindications**
It is contraindicated in cases of diarrhea due to damp-heat or food stagnation.

■ **Modern Applications**
Chronic enteritis, intestinal tuberculosis, chronic illness or elderly diarrhea, etc.

Si Sheng Wan-Four Fresh Pill
Pills of Four Fresh Ingredients
四生丸

■ **Ingredients**

Sheng He Ye	Lotus Leaf	9g
Sheng Ai Ye	Mugwort Leaf	9g
Sheng Ce Bai Ye	Biota Leaf	12g
Sheng Di Huang	Dried Rehmannia	15g

■ **Preparation**
Use as decoction or prepared form. All ingredients are used as fresh.

■ **Pertaining Category**
Stopping Bleeding

■ **Functions**
Cools blood, stops bleeding.

■ **Indications**
Mild heat in the blood affecting the upper and middle burners manifested as all kinds of bleeding such as vomiting of blood, nosebleeding with fresh red colored blood, dry mouth and throat, red or dark red tongue, a wiry, rapid pulse.

■ **Cautions and Contraindications**
None noted.

■ **Modern Applications**
Epistaxis, hematemesis, hemoptysis, peptic ulcer, acute gastritis, bronchiectasis, gingivitis, etc.
This formula is mild than Shi Hui San (Ten Charred Ingredients Powder).

Si Wu Tang-Four Substances Decoction
Tang-kuei Four Combination
四 物 汤

■ **Ingredients**

Dang Gui	Chinese Angelica	10g
Shu Di Huang	Cooked Rehmannia	12g
Bai Shao Yao	White Peony	12g
Chuan Xiong	Ligusticum	8g

■ **Preparation**
Use as decoction or prepared form.

■ **Pertaining Category**
Blood Tonifying

■ **Functions**
Nourishes blood, harmonizes blood circulation, benefits the liver.

■ **Indications**
Deficiency of blood manifested as dizziness, blurred vision, pale complexion, pale lips and nails, numbness of limbs, irregular menstruation with scanty flow, abdominal pain or uterine bleeding, restless fetus due to lack of nourishment, pale tongue, a thin, weak, and hesitant pulse.

■ **Cautions and Contraindications**
It is contraindicated in cases of poor appetite, diarrhea due to spleen Yang deficiency.

■ **Modern Applications**
Anemia, irregular menstruation, amenorrhea, threatened abortion, postpartum anemia, neurasthenia, malnutrition, etc.

Su He Xiang Wan-Styrax Pill
Styrax Formula
苏 合 香 丸

■ Ingredients

Su He Xiang	*Styrax*	30g
Qing Mu Xiang	*Aristolochia*	60g
Xiang Fu	*Cyperus Tuber*	60g
Tan Xiang	*Santalum*	60g
An Xi Xiang	*Benzoin*	60g
Chen Xiang	*Aquilaria*	60g
She Xiang	*Musk*	60g
Ding Xiang	*Cloves*	60g
Ru Xiang	*Frankincense*	30g
Bing Pian	*Borneol*	30g
Xi Jiao	*Rhinoceros Horn*	60g
Bai Zhu	*White Atractylodes*	60g
Bi Ba	*Long Pepper*	60g
Zhu Sha	*Cinnabar*	60g
He Zi	*Myrobalan Fruit*	60g

■ Preparation
Use as prepared form.

■ Pertaining Category
Aromatically Opening Orifices with Warm Nature

■ Functions
Opens orifices aromatically, induces resuscitation. Resolves cold phlegm. Moves Qi circulation, relieves pain.

■ Indications
Cold phlegm-dampness misting the heart orifice manifested as sudden fainting, clenched jaw, loss of consciousness, fullness and coldness in the chest and abdomen, chest or abdominal pain, nausea, feeling of urge to vomit, cold hands and feet, whitish face, cold oral and nasal breath, pale and moist tongue with white coat, a deep, slow, and forceful or wiry, tight, and forceful pulse.

■ Cautions and Contraindications
It is contraindicated for pregnant woman or coma due to phlegm-heat. Do not use overdose and for long term.

■ Modern Applications
Stroke, epilepsy, coronary heart disease, angina pectoris, hysterical syncope, etc.

Su Ye Huang Lian Tang-Perilla Leaf and Coptis Decoction
Perilla Leaf and Coptis Combination
苏叶黄连汤

■ Ingredients

| Zi Su Ye | *Perilla Leaf* | 9g |
| Huang Lian | *Coptis* | 9g |

■ Preparation
Use as decoction or prepared form.

■ Pertaining Category
Additional Formulas for Ob-Gyn Disorders

■ Functions
Soothes the liver, harmonizes the stomach. Descends rebellious Qi, stops vomiting.

■ Indications
Morning sickness due to disharmony between the liver and stomach manifested as vomiting of acid or bitter fluids during early pregnancy, a fullness sensation in the chest, hypochondriac pain, frequent sighing and belching, a distending sensation of head with dizziness, irritability, thirst, a bitter taste in the mouth, light red tongue with yellowish coat, a wiry, slippery pulse.

322

Cautions and Contraindications

None noted.

Modern Applications

Morning sickness, gastric neurosis, etc.

For best results, the following herbs can be added: Ban Xia(Pinellia Tuber)9g, Chen Pi(Tangerine Peel)9g, Zhu Ru(Bamboo Shavings)9g, Wu Mei(Black Plum)6g.

Su Zi Jiang Qi Tang-Perilla Seed Descending Qi Decoction
Perilla Fruit Decoction
苏子降气汤

Ingredients

Zi Su Zi	Perilla Seed	9g
Ban Xia	Pinellia Tuber	9g
Dang Gui	Chinese Angelica	6g
Qian Hu	Hogfennel Root	6g
Hou Po	Magnolia Bark	6g
Rou Gui	Cinnamon Bark	3g
Zhi Gan Cao	Baked Licorice	6g
Zi Su Ye	Perilla Leaf	2g
Sheng Jiang	Fresh Ginger	2slices
Da Zao	Jujube	1pc

Preparation

Use as decoction or prepared form.

Pertaining Category

Qi Regulating(Descending)

Functions

Descends rebellious Qi, relieves asthma. Resolves cold phlegm, stops coughing.

323

Indications

Phlegm-damp in the lungs with Qi and Yang deficiency in the kidney manifested as cough with wheezing and profuse sputum, shortness of breath worsen with exertion, a fullness sensation or pain in the cheat, soreness and weakness in the lower back and lower limbs, lassitude, dizziness, or edema, pale tongue with white greasy and moist coat, a weak, slippery pulse.

■ Cautions and Contraindications

It is improper to use this formula for asthma due to both lung and kidney deficiency or phlegm-heat in the lungs.

■ Modern Applications

Chronic bronchitis, bronchial asthma, emphysema, pulmonary heart disease, etc.

Suan Zao Ren Tang-Wild Jujube Seed Decoction
Zizyphus Combination
酸枣仁汤

■ Ingredients

Suan Zao Ren	Zizyphus	15-18g
Zhi Mu	Anemarrhena	8-10g
Fu Ling	Hoelen/Poria	10g
Chuan Xiong	Ligusticum	3-5g
Gan Cao	Licorice	3g

■ Preparation

Use as decoction or prepared form.

■ Pertaining Category

Spirit Calming with Nourishing Sedative Herbs

■ Functions
Nourishes blood, calms spirit. Clears heat, relieves irritability.

■ Indications
Deficiency of the liver blood and Yin failing to nourish the heart manifested as insomnia, palpitation, irritability, dizziness, blurred vision, night sweats, dry mouth and throat, pale or red tongue with thin coat, a wiry, thin, or rapid pulse.

■ Cautions and Contraindications
None noted.

■ Modern Applications
Insomnia, neurasthenia, cardiac neurosis, paroxysmal tachycardia, menopausal syndrome, etc.

Suo Quan Wan-Reduce Stream Pill
Lindera and Black Cardamon Combination
缩 泉 丸

■ Ingredients

Wu Yao	Lindera Root	9-12g
Yi Zhi Ren	Alpinia	9-12g
Shan Yao	Dioscorea	9-15g

■ Preparation
Use as decoction or prepared form.

■ Pertaining Category
Binding the Essence to Stop Seminal Emission and Enuresis

■ Functions
Warms the kidney, dispels cold, treats enuresis.

■ Indications

Deficiency of the kidney Qi and Yang manifested as frequent and clear urination, enuresis, spermatorrhea, leukorrhea, pale tongue with white coat, a deep, frail pulse.

■ Cautions and Contraindications

None noted.

■ Modern Applications

Enuresis, leukorrhea, spermatorrhea, etc.

Tai Shan Pan Shi San-Mount Tai Stabilizing Powder

Treat Threatened Abortion Powder

泰山磐石散

■ Ingredients

Ren Shen	Ginseng	5g
Huang Qi	Astragalus	15g
Dang Gui	Chinese Angelica	8g
Xu Duan	Teasel Root	5g
Huang Qin	Scute	5g
Bai Zhu	White Atractylodes	10g
Chuan Xiong	Ligusticum	4g
Bai Shao Yao	White Peony	6g
Shu Di Huang	Cooked Rehmannia	10g
Sha Ren	Amomum Fruit	4g
Zhi Gan Cao	Baked Licorice	4g
Nuo Mi	Glutinous Rice	5g

■ Preparation

Use as decoction or prepared form.

■ Pertaining Category

Qi and Blood Tonifying

■ **Functions**

Tonifies Qi, strengthens spleen. Nourishes blood, calms fetus to prevent miscarriage.

■ **Indications**

Pregnant woman with Qi and blood deficiency manifested as restless fetus, lower abdominal pain, light red colored bleeding, pale complexion, malaise, poor appetite, or with history of miscarriage, pale tongue with thin white coat, a deep, weak, and slippery pulse.

■ **Cautions and Contraindications**

The formula needs to be modified if the threatened abortion is caused by heat.

■ **Modern Applications**

Threatened miscarriage, habitual abortion.
For pregnant woman with history of miscarriage, it is usually taken once a week from the second to the forth month of pregnancy.

Tai Yuan Yin-Fetal Origin Beverage
胎 元 饮

■ **Ingredients**

Ren Shen	Ginseng	9g
Dang Gui	Chinese Angelica	6g
Du Zhong	Eucommia Bark	12g
Bai Shao Yao	White Peony	12g
Shu Di Huang	Cooked Rehmannia	12g
Bai Zhu	White Atractylodes	12g
Chen Pi	Tangerine Peel	6g
Zhi Gan Cao	Baked Licorice	6g

■ **Preparation**

Use as decoction or prepared form.

■ Pertaining Category
Additional Formulas for Ob-Gyn Disorders

■ Functions
Tonifies Qi, nourishes blood. Strengthens the kidneys, calms the fetus.

■ Indications
Threatened miscarriage due to deficiency of Qi and blood manifested as slight vaginal bleeding with pale red color and thin quality during pregnancy, pain in the lower back and lower abdomen with a bearing down sensation, pale complexion, fatigue, palpitation, shortness of breath, pale tongue with thin white coat, a thin, slippery pulse.

■ Cautions and Contraindications
None noted.

■ Modern Applications
Threatened miscarriage, habitual abortion, premature delivery, anemia, etc.

Tao He Cheng Qi Tang-Persica Seed Decoction for Purging Down Digestive Qi
Persica and Rhubarb Combination
桃核承气汤

■ Ingredients

Tao Ren	Peach Kernel	12-15g
Da Huang	Rhubarb	12g
Mang Xiao	Mirabilitum	6g
Gui Zhi	Cinnamon Twig	6g
Zhi Gan Cao	Baked Licorice	6g

■ Preparation
Use as decoction or prepared form.

■ Pertaining Category
Blood Invigorating

■ Functions
Breaks up blood stasis. Eliminates heat.

■ Indications
Blood stasis with heat in the lower burner manifested as sudden abdominal pain, menstrual cramps, or amenorrhea, constipation with dark colored stools, irritability, thirst, or even delirium, mania, fever at night, red and dry or purple tongue, a deep, forceful, and hesitant pulse.

■ Cautions and Contraindications
It is contraindicated during pregnancy and in cases of exterior patterns.

■ Modern Applications
Irregular menstruation, amenorrhea, dysmenorrhea, endometriosis, pelvic inflammatory disease, retention of placenta, incomplete intestinal obstruction, etc.

Tao Hong Si Wu Tang-Four Substances Decoction with Peach Kernel and Safflower
桃 红 四 物 汤

■ Ingredients

Shu Di Huang	Cooked Rehmannia	12-15g
Dang Gui	Chinese Angelica	12g
Bai Shao Yao	White Peony	10g
Chuan Xiong	Ligusticum	8g
Tao Ren	Peach Kernel	6g
Hong Hua	Safflower	4g

■ **Preparation**
Use as decoction or prepared form.

■ **Pertaining Category**
Blood Tonifying

■ **Functions**
Nourishes blood. Promotes blood circulation, removes blood stasis.

■ **Indications**
Blood deficiency with mild blood stagnation manifested as
shortened menstrual cycle, dark purple bleeding and thick quality
with or without clots, lower abdominal distention and pain, or chest
pain, or pain due to traumatic injury, pale or purple tongue, a wiry,
thin, and hesitant pulse.

■ **Cautions and Contraindications**
It is contraindicated during pregnancy.

■ **Modern Applications**
Irregular menstruation, dysmenorrhea, antedated menstruation,
angina pectoris, trauma, etc.

Tao Hua Tang-Peach Blossom Decoction
Peach Blossom Formula
桃花汤

■ **Ingredients**

Chi Shi Zhi	Halloysite	30g
Gan Jiang	Dried Ginger	9g
Geng Mi	Oryza	30g

■ **Preparation**
Use as decoction or prepared form.

■ **Pertaining Category**
Astringing the Intestines to Stop Diarrhea

■ Functions

Warms the middle burner, tonifies the spleen, astringes the intestines.

■ Indications

Deficient cold in the spleen and stomach manifested as chronic dysentery with dark blood and pus in the stools, abdominal pain which is alleviated by pressure and warmth, cold limbs, difficult urination, pale tongue, a slow and frail, or thin, faint pulse.

■ Cautions and Contraindications

None noted.

■ Modern Applications

Chronic dysentery, chronic colitis, ulcerative colitis, peptic ulcer, Crohn's disease, hemorrhoids, etc.

Tao Ren Hong Hua Jian-Peach Kernel and Safflower Brew
Persica and Safflower Combination
桃仁红花煎

■ Ingredients

Tao Ren	Peach Kernel	9g
Hong Hua	Safflower	9g
Dan Shen	Salvia Root	12g
Chi Shao Yao	Red Peony	9g
Chuan Xiong	Ligusticum	6g
Yan Hu Suo	Corydalis	9g
Xiang Fu	Cyperus Tuber	6g
Qing Pi	Green Citrus Peel	6g
Sheng Di Huang	Dried Rehmannia	9g
Dang Gui	Chinese Angelica	9g

■ **Preparation**

Use as decoction or prepared form.

■ **Pertaining Category**

Blood Invigorating

■ **Functions**

Invigorates blood, moves Qi, removes blood stasis, unblocks channels and collaterals.

■ **Indications**

Stagnation of heart blood with restrained liver Qi manifested as palpitation, a fullness sensation in the chest or chest pain, distending pain in the hypochondrium, purplish discoloration of the nails and lips, dark purple tongue with purplish spots, a hesitant, thin, or intermittent pulse.

■ **Cautions and Contraindications**

It is contraindicated in cases of any bleeding disorders or during pregnancy.

■ **Modern Applications**

Angina pectoris, primary or secondary dysmenorrhea, amenorrhea, traumatic arthritis, trauma, etc.

Tian Ma Gou Teng Yin-Gastrodia and Uncaria Beverage
Gastrodia and Uncaria Combination
天 麻 钩 藤 饮

■ Ingredients

Tian Ma	Gastrodia	9g
Gou Teng	Uncaria	12g
Shi Jue Ming	Abalone	18g
Zhi Zi	Gardenia Fruit	9g
Huang Qin	Scute	9g
Niu Xi	Cyathula Root	12g
Du Zhong	Eucommia Bark	9g
Yi Mu Cao	Motherwort	9g
Sang Ji Sheng	Loranthus	9g
Ye Jiao Teng	Fleeceflower Stem	9g
Fu Shen	Hoelen/Poria	9g

■ Preparation

Use as decoction or prepared form. Shi Jue Ming should be decocted prior to other herbs. Gou Teng should be added near the end.

■ Pertaining Category

Internal Wind Extinguishing

■ Functions

Subdues the liver Yang, extinguishes wind. Clears heat, calms the spirit. Promotes blood circulation. Nourishes the liver and kidneys.

■ Indications

Liver Yang raising or liver wind stirring up with disturbance of spirit manifested as headache, dizziness, blurred vision, tinnitus, irritability, easy to get angry, palpitation, insomnia, trembling of hands and feet, numbness of limbs, or even hemiplegia with deviated mouth and eyes, red tongue, a wiry, thin, and rapid pulse.

■ Cautions and Contraindications
None noted.

■ Modern Applications
Hypertension, cerebrovascular accident, epilepsy, vertigo, hyperthyroidism, dysfunction of vegetative (autonomic) nerve, menopausal syndrome, etc.

Tian Tai Wu Yao San-Heaven Stage Lindera Powder
Top Quality Lindera Powder
天 台 乌 药 散

■ Ingredients

Wu Yao	*Lindera*	12g
Mu Xiang	*Saussurea*	6g
Xiao Hui Xiang	*Fennel Fruit*	6g
Qing Pi	*Green Citrus Peel*	6g
Gao Liang Jiang	*Galanga*	9g
Bing Lang	*Betel Nut*	9g
Chuan Lian Zi	*Melia*	12g
Ba Dou	*Croton Seed*	70pcs

■ Preparation
Use as decoction or prepared form. Ba Dou (Croton Seed) and Chua Lian Zi (Melia) should be dry-fried together for 5-10 minutes, then discard Ba Dou and mix Chuan Lian Zi with other ingredients.

■ Pertaining Category
Qi Regulating(Moving)

■ Functions
Promotes the circulation of liver Qi, dispels cold, stops pain.

■ **Indications**

Qi stagnation of the liver channel due to cold invasion manifested as pain in the lower lateral abdomen that radiates to the genital region, testicle pain and swelling in man, or clear vaginal discharge in woman, pale tongue with white coat, a deep, slow, and wiry pulse.

■ **Cautions and Contraindications**

It is contraindicated for patients with weak constitution.

■ **Modern Applications**

Inguinal hernia, scortal hernia, leukorrhea, etc.

Tian Wang Bu Xin Dan-Heavenly Emperor Heart-Tonifying Elixir
Ginseng and Zizypghus Formula
天王补心丹

■ **Ingredients**

Sheng Di Huang	Dried Rehmannia	120g
Xuan Shen	Scrophularia	15g
Mai Men Dong	Ophiopogon	60g
Tian Men Dong	Asparagus	60g
Dang Gui	Chinese Angelica	60g
Dan Shen	Salvia	15g
Suan Zao Ren	Zizyphus	60g
Bai Zi Ren	Biota Seed	60g
Ren Shen	Ginseng	15g
Fu Ling	Hoelen/Poria	15g
Yuan Zhi	Polygala	15g
Wu Wei Zi	Schizandra	15g
Jie Geng	Platycodon	15g
Zhu Sha	Cinnabar	9-15g

■ **Preparation**

Use as prepared form or decoction with properly reduced dosage.

■ **Pertaining Category**

Spirit Calming with Nourishing Sedative Herbs

■ **Functions**

Nourishes Yin, clears deficient heat. Tonifies the heart blood and Qi, calms spirit.

■ **Indications**

Yin and blood deficiency of the heart and kidney with deficient fire flaring-up disturbing spirit manifested as irritability, insomnia, palpitation, mental fatigue, forgetfulness, dream disturbed sleep with nocturnal emission, night sweats, dry stools, ulceration on the tongue, red tongue with scanty coat, a thin, rapid pulse.

■ **Cautions and Contraindications**

Do not use overdose and for long term. Do not use during pregnancy. Use with caution for patients with a weak digestive system.

■ **Modern Applications**

Neurasthenia, paroxysmal tachycardia, hypertension, hyperthyroidism, etc.

Tiao Wei Cheng Qi Tang-Regulate Stomach Decoction for Purging Down Digestive Qi
Rhubarb and Mirabilitum Combination
调胃承气汤

■ **Ingredients**

Da Huang	Rhubarb	12g
Mang Xiao	Mirabilitum	12g
Gan Cao	Licorice	6g

■ Preparation

Use as decoction or prepared form. Mang Xiao (Mirabilitum) should be infused in the decoction just before the oral dose.

■ Pertaining Category

Purging Downward with Cold Nature

■ Functions

Relieves pathogenic heat accumulation by mildly and slowly purging effect. Regulates the stomach.

■ Indications

Mild case of heat accumulating in the Yangming Fu organ manifested as constipation, thirst, irritability, fever, abdominal distention, or delirium, or excessive heat causing rashes, vomiting of blood, nose bleeding, toothache, sore throat, yellow tongue coat, a slippery, rapid pulse.

■ Cautions and Contraindications

It is contraindicated in cases of patients with weak constitution, exterior patterns, and women during pregnancy. It should be discontinued immediately after the bowel has moved.

■ Modern Applications

Constipation, acute simple intestinal obstruction, acute appendicitis, acute cholecystitis, mouth sores, gingivitis, etc.

Ting Li Da Zao Xie Fei Tang-Drain the Lung Decoction with Lepidium and Jujube
Lepidium and Jujube Combination
葶 苈 大 枣 泻 肺 汤

■ Ingredients

| Ting Li Zi | Lepidium | 10-15g |
| Da Zao | Jujube | 12pcs |

- **Preparation**

Use as decoction or prepared form.

- **Pertaining Category**

Clearing Heat from Zang-fu Organs

- **Functions**

Drains phlegm-fluid from the lungs. Descends the lung Qi, relieves coughing and wheezing.

- **Indications**

Phlegm-fluid accumulating in the lungs or lung abscess with phlegm manifested as cough and wheezing with excessive sputum, fullness in the chest, edema of face and eyes, or difficulty in urination, white greasy tongue coat, a slippery, pulse.

- **Cautions and Contraindications**

Use with extreme caution for weak constitution patients.

- **Modern Applications**

Asthma, chronic bronchitis, pneumonia, pleural effusion, cardiac edema, etc.

Tong Mai Si Ni Tang-Unblock the Channels Decoction for Four Frigid Limbs
Licorice, Aconite, and Ginger Pulse Combination
通 脉 四 逆 汤

- **Ingredients**

Gan Jiang	*Dried Ginger*	9g
Zhi Gan Cao	*Baked Licorice*	6g
Sheng Fu Zi	*Aconite*	1big piece (12-15g)

■ **Preparation**
Use as decoction. Sheng Fu Zi should be decocted first for one hour.

■ **Pertaining Category**
Rescuing Collapsed Yang

■ **Functions**
Rescues Yang, unblocks channel, restores the pulse.

■ **Indications**
Shaoyin syndrome of true cold with false heat floating to the exterior manifested as cold limbs upon touch but no intolerance to cold, flushed face, diarrhea with undigested food in the stools, or vomiting, pale or light purple tongue with toothmarks and thin white coat, a faint or hidden pulse that is almost imperceptible.

■ **Cautions and Contraindications**
It is contraindicated in cases of cold limbs due to interior accumulation of heat. For patients with flushed face due to true cold and false heat, the formula should be taken in cool.

■ **Modern Applications**
Chronic consumptive disease, hypopituitarism, hypothyroidism, hypoadrenocorticism, shock due to heart failure or cardiac infarction, chronic gastroenteritis, cholera, gastroptosis, chronic dysentery, blood loss, dehydration, etc.
This formula is used for more serious condition than that for which the Si Ni Tang is used, because of increased dosage of Fu Zi and Gan Jiang, especially for relatively severe heart Yang deficiency.

Tong Qiao Huo Xue Tang-Unblock the Orifices and Move Blood Decoction
Persica and Cnidium Combination
通 窍 活 血 汤

■ Ingredients

Chi Shao Yao	Red Peony	3g
Chuan Xiong	Ligusticum	3g
Tao Ren	Peach Kernel	9g
Hong Hua	Safflower	9g
Cong Bai	Allium Bulb	3g
Da Zao	Jujube	5-7pcs
Sheng Jiang	Fresh Ginger	6g
She Xiang	Musk	0.1-0.3g
Huang Jiou	Rice Wine	proper amount

■ Preparation

Use as decoction or prepared form.

■ Pertaining Category

Blood Invigorating

■ Functions

Promotes blood circulation, removes blood stasis, unblocks the orifices.

■ Indications

Blood stasis in the head and face manifested as headache with pricking pain and fixed location, dizziness, prolonged deafness, or loss of hair, dark complexion, or with rosacea, or childhood malnutrition with emaciation, abdominal distention, tidal fever due to stasis, or female blood exhaustion with blood stasis, purple tongue with purplish spots, a wiry, hesitant pulse.

340

■ **Cautions and Contraindications**

It is contraindicated during pregnancy and in cases of excessive menstrual bleeding, bleeding diathesis, or any bleeding disorders, etc.

■ **Modern Applications**

Prolonged headache due to trauma, cerebral concussion, sequela of cerebral concussion, infantile malnutrition, amenorrhea, rosacea, vitiligo, etc.

Tong Ru Dan-Promote Lactation Elixir
通乳丹

■ **Ingredients**

Ren Shen	Ginseng	9g
Huang Qi	Astragalus	18g
Dang Gui	Chinese Angelica	12g
Mai Men Dong	Ophiopogon	9g
Mu Tong	Akebia	6g
Jie Geng	Platycodon	6g

■ **Preparation**

Use as decoction or prepared form. Decocts above herbs in a soup of pig feet.

■ **Pertaining Category**

Additional Formulas for Ob-Gyn Disorders

■ **Functions**

Tonifies Qi, nourishes blood, promotes lactation.

Indications

Insufficient lactation due to deficiency of Qi and blood manifested as insufficiency or complete cessation of milk secretion after delivery, soft breasts without distention, lusterless complexion, listlessness, fatigue, poor appetite, loose stools, pale tongue with little coat, a thin, weak pulse.

Cautions and Contraindications

Do not use overdose and for long term.

Modern Applications

Insufficient lactation, etc.

Tong Xie Yao Fang-Important Formula for Painful Diarrhea
Siler and Atractylodes Formula
痛 泻 要 方

Ingredients

Bai Zhu	White Atractylodes	90g
Bai Shao Yao	White Peony	60g
Chen Pi	Tangerine Peel	45g
Fang Feng	Siler	60g

Preparation

Use as prepared form or decoction with properly reduced dosage.

Pertaining Category

Regulating the Liver and Spleen (Mediating)

Functions

Disperses liver Qi, relieves abdominal pain. Strengthens spleen, stops diarrhea.

■ Indications

Disharmony between the liver and spleen manifested as recurrent abdominal pain, borborygmus, diarrhea, abdominal pain is not alleviated after bowel movement, thin white tongue coat, a wiry, slow, thin pulse.

■ Cautions and Contraindications

None noted.

■ Modern Applications

Enteritis, allergic colitis, children's indigestion, etc.

Tou Nong San-Discharge Pus Powder
The Pustulant Powder
透 脓 散

■ Ingredients

Huang Qi	Astragalus	12g
Dang Gui	Chinese Angelica	6g
Chuan Shan Jia	Pangolin Scales	3g
Zao Jiao Ci	Gleditsia	4.5g
Chuan Xiong	Ligusticum	9g

■ Preparation

Use as decoction, taken with yellow rice wine.

■ Pertaining Category

Treating External Carbuncles

■ Functions

Tonifies Qi, nourishes blood. Expels toxins, promotes pus discharge.

■ **Indications**

Chronic carbuncles and boils with deficiency of Qi and blood manifested as formed pus stays trapped under the skin and is not easy to break and discharge, accompanied by local warmth, pain, and swelling, shortness of breath, lassitude, poor appetite, pale tongue with thin white coat, a weak, thin pulse.

■ **Cautions and Contraindications**

It is contraindicated during pregnancy.

■ **Modern Applications**

Carbuncles with formation of pus or deep-rooted boils that is not easy to ulcerate, abscess, bone tuberculosis, etc.

This formula is from "Wai Ke Zheng Zong"(True Lineage of External Medicine). With additional ingredients (Bai Zhi, Niu Bang Zi, Jin Yin Hua) is also known as Tou Nong San, which is from "Yi Xue Xin Wu"(Medical Revelation). The latter has stronger effect of discharging pus.

Wan Dai Tang-End Discharge Decoction
Cease Leukorrhea Decoction
完带汤

■ **Ingredients**

Bai Zhu	White Atractylodes	30g
Shan Yao	Dioscorea	30g
Ren Shen	Ginseng	6g
Bai Shao Yao	White Peony	15g
Che Qian Zi	Plantago Seed	9g
Cang Zhu	Atractylodes	9g
Chen Pi	Tangerine Peel	1.5g
Jing Jie Sui	Schizonepeta Spike	1.5g
Chai Hu	Bupleurum	1.8g
Gan Cao	Licorice	3g

■ Preparation

Use as decoction or prepared form. Che Qian Zi should be wrapped in gauze when making decoction.

■ Pertaining Category

Stabilizing the Menses and Stopping Leukorrhea

■ Functions

Tonifies the spleen, transforms dampness, stops leukorrhea.

■ Indications

Spleen Qi deficiency and liver Qi stagnation with dampness retention manifested as white, watery, thin vaginal discharge without bad odor, pale complexion, lassitude, loose stools, poor appetite, pale tongue with white coat, a soft, weak pulse.

■ Cautions and Contraindications

It is contraindicated in cases of leukorrhea due to damp-heat.

■ Modern Applications

Leukorrhea, inflammation of the genital system, vaginitis, etc.

Wei Jing Tang-Reed Decoction
Phragmites Combination
苇茎汤

■ Ingredients

Lu Gen	Reed Rhizome	30g
Yi Yi Ren	Coix Seed	30g
Dong Gua Ren	Benincasa	24g
Tao Ren	Peach Kernel	9g

■ Preparation

Use as decoction or prepared form.

■ **Pertaining Category**
Treating Internal Abscess

■ **Functions**
Clears the lung heat, resolves phlegm. Removes blood stasis, promotes pus discharge.

■ **Indications**
Toxic phlegm-heat and stagnant blood in the lungs manifested as cough with blood streaked thick, yellow, and foul smelling sputum or with bloody pus, mild chest pain that is aggravated by coughing, or fever, dry and squamous skin, red tongue with yellow greasy coat, a slippery, rapid pulse.

■ **Cautions and Contraindications**
It is contraindicated during pregnancy.

■ **Modern Applications**
Pulmonary abscess, pneumonia, bronchitis, whooping cough, measles, bronchiectasis, etc.

Wei Ling Tang-Stomach-calming and Hoelen Five Decoction
Decoction to Dispel Dampness in the Spleen and Stomach
胃苓汤

■ Ingredients

Ze Xie	Alisma Tuber	12g
Fu Ling	Hoelen/Poria	9g
Zhu Ling	Polyporus	9g
Bai Zhu	White Atractylodes	9g
Gui Zhi	Cinnamon Twig	6g
Cang Zhu	Atractylodes	12g
Hou Po	Magnolia Bark	9g
Chen Pi	Tangerine Peel	9g
Gan Cao	Licorice	4g
Sheng Jiang	Fresh Ginger	3slices
Da Zao	Jujube	2pcs

■ Preparation

Use as decoction or prepared form.

■ Pertaining Category

Downward Dampness Draining

■ Functions

Dispels dampness, regulates Qi in the middle burner. Strengthens the spleen, harmonizes the stomach.

■ Indications

Dampness accumulating in the middle burner manifested as epigastric and abdominal distention, poor appetite, watery diarrhea, general heaviness of the body, difficult urination, or edema, white greasy tongue coat, a slippery, soft, and thin pulse.

■ Cautions and Contraindications

It is contraindicated for patients with Yin deficiency.

■ Modern Applications

Chronic gastritis, enteritis, gastric neurosis, cardiac and nephritic edema, ascites, retention of urine, etc.

This formula is a combination of Ping Wei San and Wu Ling San.

Wen Dan Tang-Warm the Gallbladder Decoction
Bamboo and Hoelen Combination
温 胆 汤

■ **Ingredients**

Ban Xia	Pinellia Tuber	6g
Zhu Ru	Bamboo Shavings	6g
Zhi Shi	Immature Citrus	6g
Chen Pi	Tangerine Peel	9g
Fu Ling	Hoelen/Poria	4.5g
Sheng Jiang	Fresh Ginger	5slices
Da Zao	Jujube	1pc
Zhi Gan Cao	Baked Licorice	3g

■ **Preparation**
Use as decoction or prepared form.

■ **Pertaining Category**
Dampness Drying and Phlegm Resolving

■ **Functions**
Regulates Qi, resolves phlegm. Clears the gallbladder, harmonizes the stomach.

■ **Indications**
Disharmony between the gallbladder and stomach with phlegm-heat manifested as irritability, insomnia, nausea, vomiting, hiccups, dizziness, palpitation, timidity, a fullness sensation in the chest, a bitter taste in the mouth, or seizures with copious foamy sputum, thin white or yellowish greasy tongue coat, a slippery pulse.

■ Cautions and Contraindications
It is contraindicated in cases of insomnia, palpitation, and
dizziness due to Yin or blood deficiency, or vomiting due to
stomach cold.

■ Modern Applications
Chronic bronchitis or trachitis, pulmonary emphysama, chronic
gastritis, peptic ulcer, chronic hepatitis, insomnia, neurosis,
epilepsy, Miniere's syndrome, early stage of schizophrenia, etc.

Wen Jing Tang-Warm the Menses Decoction
Tang-kuei and Evodia Combination
温 经 汤

■ Ingredients

Dang Gui	*Chinese Angelica*	9g
Wu Zhu Yu	*Evodia*	9g
Bai Shao Yao	*White Peony*	6g
Chuan Xiong	*Ligusticum*	6g
Ren Shen	*Ginseng*	6g
Gui Zhi	*Cinnamon Twig*	6g
E Jiao	*Equus/Gelatin*	6-9g
Mu Dan Pi	*Moutan Bark*	6g
Ban Xia	*Pinellia Tuber*	6g
Mai Men Dong	*Ophiopogon*	9g
Sheng Jiang	*Fresh Ginger*	6g
Gan Cao	*Licorice*	6g

■ Preparation
Use as decoction or prepared form. E Jiao should be dissolved
separately in boiling water and added into the strained decoction.

■ Pertaining Category
Blood Invigorating

■ Functions
Warms the channels and uterus, dispels cold. Removes blood stasis.
Nourishes blood.

■ Indications
Deficient cold in the Chong and Ren channels with blood stasis and
insufficient blood and Yin manifested as prolonged menstrual
duration, or spotting between periods, irregular menstruation,
coldness, pain, and fullness in the lower abdomen, or lower grade
fever at night, a feverish sensation in the palms, dry mouth and lips,
or difficult to conceive, pale, purplish tongue or with purple spots, a
deep, wiry, and slow pulse.

■ Cautions and Contraindications
None noted.

■ Modern Applications
Irregular menstruation, amenorrhea, dysmenrrhea, functional uterine
bleeding, infertility, polycystic ovaries, chronic pelvic
inflammation, etc.
*This condition is complicated with cold and heat, deficient and
excess.*

Wen Pi Tang-Warm the Spleen Decoction
Rhubarb and Ginger Combination
温脾汤

■ Ingredients

Da Huang	Rhubarb	12g
Fu Zi	Prepared Aconite	9g
Gan Jiang	Dried Ginger	6g
Ren Shen	Ginseng	6g
Gan Cao	Licorice	6g

■ Preparation
Use as decoction. Fu Zi (Prepared Aconite) should be decocted 30-60 minutes prior to other herbs; Da Huang (Rhubarb) should be added later.

■ Pertaining Category
Purging Downward with Warm Nature

■ Functions
Warms and tonifies the Spleen Yang. Purges bowel movement, eliminates cold accumulation.

■ Indications
Accumulation of deficient cold due to spleen Yang deficiency manifested as constipation or dysentery, abdominal cold pain around the umbilicus, which is alleviated by warmth and pressure, epigastric fullness, cold limbs, pale tongue with white coat, a deep, wiry pulse.

■ Cautions and Contraindications
It is contraindicated during pregnancy.

■ Modern Applications
Constipation, chronic appendicitis, chronic gastritis, chronic enteritis, chronic dysentery, chronic ulcerative colitis, intestinal tuberculosis, simple intestinal obstruction, uremia, etc.

Wu Bi Shan Yao Wan-Matchless Chinese Wild Yam Pill
Dioscorea Pill
无 比 山 药 丸

Ingredients

Shan Yao	*Dioscorea*	30g
Rou Cong Rong	*Cistanche*	15g
Shu Di Huang	*Cooked Rehmannia*	12g
Shan Zhu Yu	*Dogwood Fruit*	12g
Fu Shen	*Hoelen/Poria*	9g
Tu Si Zi	*Dodder Seed*	9g
Wu Wei Zi	*Schisandra*	6g
Chi Shi Zhi	*Halloysite*	9g
Ba Ji Tian	*Morinda Root*	12g
Ze Xie	*Alisma*	9g
Du Zhong	*Eucommia Bark*	12g
Huai Niu Xi	*Achyranthes Root*	9g

Preparation

Use as decoction or prepared form.

Pertaining Category

Yang Tonifying

Functions

Warms the kidney Yang, strengthens spleen, benefits urinary system.

Indications

Chronic urinary strangury due to Qi and Yang deficiency of the kidney and spleen manifested as urine not quite difficult and dark, but periodically involuntary dribbing which usually get worse after exertion, soreness and weakness of lower back, lassitude, pale tongue, a weak pulse.

Cautions and Contraindications

None noted.

Modern Applications

Chronic nephritis, chronic urethritis, diabetes, etc.

Wu Ling San-Five Ingredients Powder with Poria

Hoelen Five Herbs Formula
五苓散

■ Ingredients

Fu Ling	Hoelen/Poria	9g
Zhu Ling	Polyporus	9g
Ze Xie	Alisma Tuber	15g
Bai Zhu	White Atractylodes	9g
Gui Zhi	Cinnamon Twig	6g

■ Preparation
Use as decoction or prepared form.

■ Pertaining Category
Downward Dampness Draining

■ Functions
Induces diuresis, drains dampness. Warms Yang, tonifies the spleen, strengthens the transforming function of Qi. Releases the exterior.

■ Indications
Water retention with spleen Qi deficiency or mild wind-cold in the exterior manifested as headache, fever, difficult urination, or vomiting after drinking water, edema, diarrhea, spitting saliva or phlegm-fluid, shortness of breath, dizziness, a feeling of palpitation below the umbilicus, white, thick, greasy tongue coat, a slippery or superficial pulse.

■ Cautions and Contraindications
It is contraindicated in cases of difficult scanty urination due to Yin deficiency.

■ Modern Applications
Acute gastroenteritis, initial stage of acute nephritis, chronic nephritis, chronic renal failure, congestive heart failure, ascites from liver cirrhosis, Meniere's syndrome, retention of urine, etc.

Wu Mei Wan-Mume Pill

Mume Formula

乌梅丸

■ Ingredients

Wu Mei	Black Plum	480g
Xi Xin	Asarum	180g
Gan Jiang	Dried Ginger	300g
Huang Lian	Coptis	480g
Dang Gui	Chinese Angelica	120g
Fu Zi	Prepared Aconite	180g
Hua Jiao	Zanthoxylum	120g
Gui Zhi	Cinnamon Twig	180g
Ren Shen	Ginseng	180g
Huang Bai	Phellodendron Bark	180g

■ Preparation

Use as prepared form or decoction with properly reduced dosage. Fu Zi should be decocted first for 30-45 minutes prior to the other ingredients.

■ Pertaining Category

Parasites Expelling

■ Functions

Warms internal organs (intestines), tonifies Qi. Calms and dispels parasites.

■ Indications

Roundworm disturbance due to upper (stomach) heat and lower (intestines) cold with deficiency of Qi and blood manifested as irritability, nausea, vomiting, or vomiting of roundworm after eating recurrent severe spasmodic abdominal pain, coldness in the hands and feet, or prolonged dysentery and diarrhea, pale tongue, a weak pulse.

354

■ **Cautions and Contraindications**
It is contraindicated in cases of diarrhea or dysentery due to damp-heat.

■ **Modern Applications**
Ascariasis, biliary ascariasis, chronic gastroenteritis, chronic dysentery, amebic dysentery, allergic colitis, etc.

Wu Mo Yin Zi-Five Milled Herb Beverage
Saussurea and Aquilaria combination
五磨饮子

■ **Ingredients**

Mu Xiang	Saussurea	6g
Chen Xiang	Aquilaria	6g
Bing Lang	Betel Nut	9g
Zhi Shi	Immature Citrus	9g
Wu Yao	Lindera	9g

■ **Preparation**
Use as decoction or prepared form.

■ **Pertaining Category**
Qi Regulating(Descending)

■ **Functions**
Moves Qi. Descends the rebellious Qi.

■ **Indications**
Qi stagnation due to severe emotional upset manifested as epigastric and abdominal distending pain, or wandering pain, light purple tongue with thin white coat, a wiry pulse.

- ■ **Cautions and Contraindications**

This formula is only used for patients with severe emotional upset and strong constitution.

- ■ **Modern Applications**

Bronchial asthma, gastritis, intestinal dysfunction, psychosis, hysteria, etc.

Wu Pi San (Yin)-Five Peel Powder (Beverage)
Hoelen and Areca Combination
五 皮 散 (饮)

- ■ **Ingredients**

Sheng Jiang Pi	Fresh Ginger Peel	9g
Sang Bai Pi	Mulberry Bark	9g
Chen Pi	Tangerine Peel	9g
Da Fu Pi	Areca Peel	9g
Fu Ling Pi	Hoelen/Poria Peel	9g

- ■ **Preparation**

Use as decoction or prepared form.

- ■ **Pertaining Category**

Downward Dampness Draining

- ■ **Functions**

Induces diuresis, drains dampness, reduces edema. Moves Qi. Strengthens the spleen.

Indications
Dampness retention with stagnant Qi and mild spleen deficiency manifested as general superficial edema, heaviness of body and limbs, a fullness sensation in the chest, epigastric and abdominal distention, shortness of breath, difficult urination, or edema during pregnancy, white greasy tongue coat, a deep, slow, and soft pulse.

■ Cautions and Contraindications
Use together with spleen-tonifying herbs for patients with severe spleen deficiency.

■ Modern Applications
Edema during pregnancy, menopausal edema, edema from protein deficiency, liver cirrhosis, congestive heart failure, initial stage of acute nephritis, etc.

Wu Ren Wan-Five Seed Pill
Apricot Seed and Prunus Formula
五仁丸

■ Ingredients

Tao Ren	Peach Kernel	15g
Xing Ren	Apricot Seed	30g
Bai Zi Ren	Biota Seed	3.75g
Yu Li Ren	Bush Cherry Seed	3g
Song Zi Ren	Pine Seed	3g
Chen Pi	Tangerine Peel	120g

■ Preparation
Use as prepared form.

■ Pertaining Category
Purging Downward with Moist Laxatives

■ Functions
Moistens the intestines, promotes bowel movement.

357

Indications

Constipation due to lack of body fluids in the intestines, elderly, postpartum, and blood deficiency, pale tongue, a thin, weak pulse.

Cautions and Contraindications

None noted.

Modern Applications

Habitual constipation, postpartum or post-surgical constipation, hemorrhoids, anal fissure, etc.

Wu Tou Tang-Aconite Decoction
Aconite and Ma-huang Combination
乌头汤

Ingredients

Ma Huang	Ephedra	6-9g
Bai Shao Yao	White Peony	9g
Huang Qi	Astragalus	9g
Zhi Gan Cao	Baked Licorice	6-9g
Zhi Chuan Wu	Prepared Sichuan Aconite	9-12g

Preparation

Use as decoction or prepared form. Zhi Chuan Wu needs to be decocted with honey for 40-60 minutes prior to the other ingredients.

Pertaining Category

Wind-dampness Expelling

Functions

Warms the channels, dispels wind-cold-dampness, alleviates pain. Replenishes Qi.

■ Indications
Wind-cold-damp bi syndrome with predominant cold and weakness of Qi manifested as severe joint pain with fixed location and cold sensation, without redness and warmth, decrease in pain with application of heat, restricted motion in the affected limbs, cold hands and feet, pale or purplish tongue with thin white coat, a wiry, tight pulse.

■ Cautions and Contraindications
Do not use for a pregnant woman or for long term.

■ Modern Applications
Rheumatic and rheumatoid arthritis, etc.

Wu Wei Xiao Du Yin-Five Ingredients Beverage to Relieve Toxin
The Antiseptic Decoction with Five-ingredients
五味消毒饮

■ Ingredients

Jin Yin Hua	Lonicera	9g
Pu Gong Ying	Dandelion	3.6g
Zi Hua Di Ding	Viola	3.6g
Tian Kuei Zi	Begonia Seed	3.6g
Ye Ju Hua	Wild Chrysanthemum	3.6g

■ Preparation
Use as decoction and taken with 1-2 tablespoons of rice wine. The herbs may be applied topically.

■ Pertaining Category
Treating External Carbuncles

■ Functions

Clears heat, relieves toxicity. Reduces swelling, softens and disperses the hard skin lesions.

■ Indications

Carbuncles, boils, and sores due to toxic fire contracted externally or produced by dysfunction of Zang-fu organs manifested as redness, swelling, burning pain, hot and hard to touch, deep rooted lesions resembling nails or chestnuts, or chills and fever, red tongue with yellow coat, rapid pulse.

■ Cautions and Contraindications

It is contraindicated in cases of carbuncle of Yin type. Use with caution for patients with spleen and stomach deficiency.

■ Modern Applications

Multiple furuncles, deep rooted boils, carbuncles, acne, erysipelas, mastitis, appendicitis, conjunctivitis, purulent osteomyelitis, pyemia, etc.

Wu Zhu Yu Tang-Evodia Decoction
Evodia Combination
吴茱萸汤

■ Ingredients

Wu Zhu Yu	Evodia	9-12g
Ren Shen	Ginseng	9g
Da Zao	Jujube	12pcs
Sheng Jiang	Fresh Ginger	18g

■ Preparation

Use as decoction or prepared form.

■ Pertaining Category

Middle Burner Warming and Cold Dispelling

■ Functions

Warms and tonifies the liver and stomach, descends the reverse flow of stomach Qi, stops vomiting.

■ Indications

Deficient cold in the middle burner affecting Jueyin and Shaoyin manifested as tendency to vomiting after eating, a stifling and fullness sensation in the chest and epigastrium, epigastric pain or discomfort with sour regurgitation, vertex headache, retching, salivation, diarrhea, cold limbs, or dysphoria, white moist tongue coat, a thin, slow, or wiry pulse.

■ Cautions and Contraindications

It is contraindicated in cases of vomiting or sour regurgitation due to heat.

■ Modern Applications

Chronic gastroenteritis, peptic ulcer, hepatitis, vomiting during pregnancy, migraine headache, Meniere's syndrome, excessive gastric acid, etc.
For patient with severe vomiting, the decoction should be taken in cool.

Wu Zi Yan Zong Wan-Five Seed Progeny Pill
Lycium and Rubus Combination
五子衍宗丸

■ Ingredients

Gou Qi Zi	Lycium Fruit	12g
Fu Pen Zi	Rubus	9g
Tu Si Zi	Dodder Seed	9g
Wu Wei Zi	Schisandra Fruit	6g
Che Qian Zi	Plantago Seed	6g

Preparation
Use as prepared form or decoction. Che Qian Zi should be wrapped in gauze when making decoction.

Pertaining Category
Additional Formulas for Internal Medicine

Functions
Warms the kidney Yang, Supplements the kidney Yin and essence.

Indications
Kidney Qi, Yang, and essence deficiency manifested as impotence, spontaneous seminal emission, infertility, frequent urination, dizziness, vertigo, tinnitus, pale complexion, cold limbs, soreness and weakness of lower back and knees, pale tongue with thin white coat, a deep, weak, and thin pulse.

Cautions and Contraindications
None noted.

Modern Applications
Infertility, impotence, elderly incontinence, spermatorrhea, chronic lower back pain, etc.

Xi Jiao Di Huang Tang-Rhinoceros Horn and Rehmannia Decoction
Rhinoceros and Rehmannia Combination
犀 角 地 黄 汤

Ingredients

Xi Jiao	Rhinoceros Horn	3g
Sheng Di Huang	Dried Rehmannia	24g
Chi Shao Yao	Red Peony	12g
Mu Dan Pi	Moutan Bark	9g

■ Preparation

Use as decoction or prepared form. Xi Jiao (Rhinoceros Horn) should be taken in powder form with strained decoction; it may be substituted by Shui Niu Jiao (Horn of the Water Buffalo) with 30g in decoction or 6g as a powder; it should be decocted separately for 15-20 minutes prior to other ingredients.

■ Pertaining Category

Ying and Blood Level Cooling

■ Functions

Clears heat from blood level, relieves toxicity. Removes blood stasis.

■ Indications

Heat penetrating into blood level resulting in various kinds of bleeding such as: vomiting of blood, nosebleeding, bloody urine or stools, dark purple color rashes, thirst without desire to drink, fever, delirium, or coma, dark red or scarlet tongue with prickles, a thin, rapid pulse.

■ Cautions and Contraindications

It is contraindicated in cases of bleeding caused by Qi deficiency and patient with deficiency of the spleen and stomach.

■ Modern Applications

Severe influenza, epidemic encephalitis B, epidemic cerebrospinal meningitis, septicemia, urimia, heptic coma, thrombocytopenic purpura, and acute leukemia, etc.

Xia Ru Yong Quan San-Promoting Lactation and Gushing Spring Powder
下乳涌泉散

Ingredients

Dang Gui	Chinese Angelica	9g
Chuan Xiong	Ligusticum	9g
Tian Hua Fen	Trichosanthes Root	9g
Bai Shao Yao	White Peony	9g
Sheng Di Huang	Dried Rehmannia	9g
Chai Hu	Bupleurum	6g
Qing Pi	Green Citrus Peel	9g
Lou Lu	Rhaponticum	9g
Jie Geng	Platycodon	6g
Tong Cao	Rice Paper Pith	6g
Bai Zhi	Angelica Root	6g
Chuan Shan Jia	Pangolin Scales	9g
Wang Bu Liu Xing	Vaccaria Seed	9g
Gan Cao	Licorice	3g

■ Preparation
Use as decoction or prepared form.

■ Pertaining Category
Additional Formulas for Ob-Gyn Disorders

■ Functions
Soothes the liver, relieves depression. Unblocks collaterals, promotes lactation.

■ Indications
Insufficient lactation due to liver Qi stagnation manifested as insufficiency or complete cessation of milk secretion after delivery, distention and pain of breasts, a fullness sensation in the chest and hypochondrium, reduced appetite, or slight fever, thin yellow tongue coat, a wiry, thin, or rapid pulse.

Cautions and Contraindications
It is contraindicated in cases of severe deficiency of Qi and blood.
Do not use overdose and for long term.

Modern Applications
Insufficient lactation, etc.

Xian Fang Huo Ming Yin-Celestial Formula for Sustaining Life Beverage
Angelica and Mastic Combination
仙方活命饮

Ingredients

Bai Zhi	Angelica Root	3g
Zhe Bei Mu	Thunberg Fritillary	3g
Fang Feng	Siler	3g
Chi Shao Yao	Red Peony	3g
Dang Gui	Chinese Angelica	3g
Zao Jiao Ci	Gleditsia	3g
Chuan Shan Jia	Pangolin Scales	3g
Tian Hua Fen	Trichosanthes Roo	3g
Ru Xiang	Frankincense	3g
Mo Yao	Myrrh	3g
Jin Yin Hua	Lonicera	9g
Chen Pi	Tangerine Peel	9g
Gan Cao	Licorice	3g

Preparation
Use as decoction. Decoct the herbs with half of water and half of wine.

Pertaining Category
Treating External Carbuncles

■ Functions
Clears heat, relieves toxicity. Reduces swelling, softens and resolves hard masses. Promotes blood circulation, stops pain.

■ Indications
Early stage of carbuncles and boils with toxic phlegm-fire and stagnation of Qi and blood manifested as redness, swelling, burning pain, fever with mild chills, red tongue with thin white or yellowish coat, a rapid, forceful pulse.

■ Cautions and Contraindications
It is contraindicated during pregnancy and in cases of carbuncle of Yin type or ulcerated carbuncles. Use with extreme caution for patients with weakness of the spleen and stomach or deficiency of Qi and blood.

■ Modern Applications
Various purulent inflammations such as multiple carbuncles, boils, ulcers, furuncle, acne, infected wounds, acute mastitis, acute purulent tonsillitis, etc.

Xiang Lian Wan-Aucklandia and Coptis Pill
Aucklandia and Coptis Formula
香 连 丸

■ Ingredients

| Mu Xiang | Saussurea | 130g |
| Huang Lian | Coptis | 60g |

■ Preparation
Fry Huang Lian (Coptis) 60g with Wu Zhu Yu (Evodia) 300g, then discard the Wu Zhu Yu (Evodia). Use as prepared form or decoction with properly reduced dosage.

■ Pertaining Category
Clearing Heat from Zang-fu Organs

366

■ Functions
Clears heat, transforms dampness. Moves Qi, relieves dysentery.

■ Indications
Dysentery or diarrhea due to damp-heat manifested as either more blood or more pus in the stools, abdominal pain with tenemus, a fullness or stifling sensation in the chest, red tongue with yellow greasy coat, a slippery, rapid pulse.

■ Cautions and Contraindications
Use with caution in cases of weakness in the spleen and stomach.

■ Modern Applications
Dysentery, acute enteritis, etc.

Xiang Ru San-Elsholtzia Powder
Elsholtzia Combination
香薷散

■ Ingredients

Xiang Ru	*Elsholtzia*	15g
Bian Dou	*Dolichos*	12g
Hou Po	*Magnolia Bark*	12g

■ Preparation
Use as decoction or prepared form.

■ Pertaining Category
Summer Heat Clearing

■ Functions
Expels summer heat and cold, releases the exterior. Transforms dampness.

■ **Indications**

Exterior cold with interior dampness in the summer manifested as fever, aversion to cold, absence of sweating, headache with heavy sensation of the head and body, a fullness sensation in the chest, nausea, or abdominal pain with vomiting and diarrhea, white greasy tongue coat, a superficial pulse.

■ **Cautions and Contraindications**

It is not advisable for patients suffering from summer heat with heat signs.

■ **Modern Applications**

Common cold in the summer, gastroenteritis, etc.

Xiang Sha Liu Jun Zi Tang-Saussurea, Amomum, and Six Gentleman Decoction
Saussurea and Cardamon Combination
香砂六君子汤

■ **Ingredients**

Ren Shen	Ginseng	9g
Bai Zhu	White Atractylodes	9g
Fu Ling	Hoelen/Poria	9g
Chen Pi	Tangerine Peel	9g
Ban Xia	Pinellia Tuber	12g
Mu Xiang	Saussurea	6g
Sha Ren	Amomum Fruit	6g
Zhi Gan Cao	Baked Licorice	6g

■ **Preparation**

Use as decoction or prepared form.

■ **Pertaining Category**

Qi Tonifying

Functions

Tonifies the spleen Qi, transforms dampness, harmonizes the stomach. Regulates Qi, alleviates pain.

Indications

Spleen and stomach Qi deficiency with dampness obstructing Qi in the middle burner manifested as poor appetite, belching, nausea, vomiting, distention and pain in the epigastric and abdominal region diarrhea, pale tongue with thin white coat, a soft, weak pulse.

Cautions and Contraindications

It is contraindicated in cases of high fever, empty fire, bloating due to food stagnation, lack of body fluid, excessive thirst, constipation. Long term use may cause thirst, dryness of tongue or mouth, and irritability.

Modern Applications

Chronic gastroenteritis, peptic ulcer, intestinal dysfunction, morning sickness, malnutrition, chronic bronchitis, etc.

Xiao Chai Hu Tang-Minor Bupleurum Decoction
Minor Bupleurum Combination
小 柴 胡 汤

Ingredients

Chai Hu	*Bupleurum*	12g
Huang Qin	*Scute*	9g
Ren Shen	*Ginseng*	6g
Ban Xia	*Pinellia Tuber*	9g
Zhi Gan Cao	*Baked Licorice*	5g
Sheng Jiang	*Fresh Ginger*	9g
Da Zao	*Jujube*	4pcs

■ **Preparation**
Use as decoction or prepared form.

■ **Pertaining Category**
Shaoyang Harmonizing (Mediating)

■ **Functions**
Harmonizes Shaoyang.

■ **Indications**
Shaoyang syndrome with pathogen located between exterior and interior manifested as alternate chills and fever, fullness and discomfort in the chest and hypochondriac region, loss of appetite, tend to vomit, irritability, a bitter taste in the mouth, blurred vision, dry throat, thin white tongue coat, a wiry pulse.

■ **Cautions and Contraindications**
It is contraindicated for patients with excess above and deficiency below, liver fire, liver Yang raising, or gum bleeding and vomiting of blood due to Yin deficiency.

■ **Modern Applications**
Common cold, woman with common cold during menstruation or after delivery, malaria, biliary tract infection, hepatitis, jaundice, pleuritis, chronic gastritis, digestive disorders, intercostal neuralgia, and AIDS, etc.

Xiao Cheng Qi Tang-Minor Decoction for Purging Down Digestive Qi
Minor Rhubarb Combination
小承气汤

■ **Ingredients**

Da Huang	*Rhubarb*	12g
Hou Po	*Magnolia Bark*	6g
Zhi Shi	*Immature Citrus*	9g

■ **Preparation**

Use as decoction or prepared form. Da Huang (Rhubarb) should be added at last 3-5 minutes when making decoction.

■ **Pertaining Category**

Purging Downward with Cold Nature

■ **Functions**

Relieves pathogenic heat accumulation by mild purging effect. Moves Qi downward.

■ **Indications**

Mild case of excessive heat accumulating in the Yangming Fu organ manifested as constipation, fullness in the chest, abdominal distention, tidal fever, delirium, red tongue with yellow or greasy coat, a rapid, slightly forceful pulse.

■ **Cautions and Contraindications**

It is contraindicated in cases of patients with weak constitution, exterior patterns, and women during pregnancy. It should be discontinued immediately after the bowel has moved.

■ **Modern Applications**

Acute appendicitis, acute cholecystitis, acute pancreatitis, acute uncomplicated intestinal obstruction, syncope, seizures, roundworm in the bile duct, early stage of dysentery, food poisoning, etc.

Xiao Er Hui Chun Dan-Children Returning Spring Elixir
小 儿 回 春 丹

- **Ingredients**

Chuan Bei Mu	Tendrilled Fritillary	37.5g
Chen Pi	Tangerine Peel	37.5g
Mu Xiang	Saussurea	37.5g
Bai Dou Kou	Cluster Fruit	37.5g
Zhi Ke	Bitter Orange	37.5g
Ban Xia	Pinellia Tuber	37.5g
Chen Xiang	Aquilaria	37.5g
Tian Zhu Huang	Bambusa	37.5g
Jiang Can	Silkworm	37.5g
Quan Xie	Scorpion	37.5g
Tan Xiang	Santalum	37.5g
Niu Huang	Ox Gallstone	12g
She Xiang	Musk	12g
Dan Nan Xing	Arisaema Tuber	60g
Gou Teng	Uncaria	24g
Da Huang	Rhubarb	60g
Tian Ma	Gastrodia	37.5g
Zhu Sha	Cinnabar	0.3-1.8g
Gan Cao	Licorice	26g

- **Preparation**

Use as prepared form.

- **Pertaining Category**

Aromatically Opening Orifices with Cold Nature

- **Functions**

Opens orifices, stops convulsion. Clears heat, resolves phlegm.

- **Indications**

Children with excessive phlegm-heat disturbing spirit and veiling the sensory orifices manifested as sudden convulsion, high fever, restlessness, vomiting of food or milk, night crying, or cough, difficulty in breathing with wheezing, or abdominal pain, diarrhea.

372

■ Cautions and Contraindications

Use with caution for children with a weak digestive system. It is contraindicated in cases of chronic convulsion due to Yang deficiency of the spleen and kidney. Do not use overdose and for long term.

■ Modern Applications

Acute infantile convulsion, toxic pneumonia or dysentery, children's epidemic encephalitis B, etc.

Xiao Feng San-Eliminate Wind Powder
Tang-kuei and Arctium Formula
消 风 散

■ Ingredients

Dang Gui	*Chinese Angelica*	3g
Sheng Di Huang	*Dried Rehmannia*	3g
Fang Feng	*Siler*	3g
Chan Tui	*Cicada Skin*	3g
Zhi Mu	*Anemarrhena*	3g
Ku Shen	*Bitter Ginseng Root*	3g
Hei Zhi Ma	*Sesame Seed*	3g
Jing Jie	*Schizonepeta*	3g
Cang Zhu	*Atractylodes*	3g
Niu Bang Zi	*Burdock Seed*	3g
Shi Gao	*Gypsum*	3g
Mu Tong	*Akebia*	1.5g
Gan Cao	*Licorice*	1.5g

■ Preparation

Use as decoction or prepared form.

■ Pertaining Category

External Wind Expelling

■ Functions
Expels wind, clears heat, eliminates dampness. Cools blood, stops itching. Nourishes blood.

■ Indications
Wind-heat and dampness invasion with pre-existing damp-heat manifested as red skin rashes with itching, spread over large part of body, exudation of the body fluid after hard scratching, red tongue with white or yellow coat, a superficial, rapid, and forceful pulse.

■ Cautions and Contraindications
It is contraindicated for patients with deficient constitution. Do not use overdose and for long term.

■ Modern Applications
Eczema, urticaria, rubella, psoriasis, contact dermatitis, etc.
This formula is from "Wai Ke Zheng Zong" (True Lineage of External Medicine).

Xiao Huo Luo Dan-Minor Invigorate the Collaterals Elixir
Sichuan and Wild Aconite Combination
小 活 络 丹

■ Ingredients

Chuan Wu Tou	Sichuan Aconite	180g
Cao Wu Tou	Wild Aconite	180g
Di Long	Earthworm	180g
Tian Nan Xing	Arisaema Tuber	180g
Ru Xiang	Frankincense	66g
Mo Yao	Myrrh	66g

■ Preparation
Use as prepared form only. Both Chuan Wu Tou and Cao Wu Tou must be prepared for taking internally.

■ **Pertaining Category**

External Wind Expelling

■ **Functions**

Expels wind-cold-dampness, transforms phlegm. Unblocks channels and collaterals, promotes blood circulation, stops pain.

■ **Indications**

Wind-cold-dampness or phlegm with blood stasis obstructing the channels and collaterals manifested as prolonged numbness of hands and feet, wandering pain in the joints with difficult movement, aching and spasms of muscles, pain and heaviness of arms, legs, and lower back, moist tongue with white coat, a slow, slippery pulse.

■ **Cautions and Contraindications**

It is contraindicated during pregnancy and for patients with weak constitution. Do not use overdose and for long term.

■ **Modern Applications**

Rheumatoid arthritis, osteoarthritis, lumbago, neck pain, shoulder pain, hemiplegia with painful limbs after cerebrovascular accident, peripheral nervous disorders, etc.

Xiao Ji Yin Zi-Small Thistle Beverage
Cephalanoplos Combination
小 蓟 饮 子

■ Ingredients

Sheng Di Huang	Dried Rehmannia	30g
Xiao Ji	Small Thistle	15g
Hua Shi	Talcum	15g
Mu Tong	Akebia	9g
Pu Huang	Cattail Pollen	9g
Ou Jie	Lotus Node	9g
Dan Zhu Ye	Bland Bamboo Leaf	9g
Dang Gui	Chinese Angelica	6g
Zhi Zi	Gardenia Fruit	9g
Zhi Gan Cao	Baked Licorice	6g

■ Preparation
Use as decoction or prepared form.

■ Pertaining Category
Stopping Bleeding

■ Functions
Cools blood, stops bleeding. Promotes urination, unblocks urinary strangury.

■ Indications
Heat accumulating in the urinary bladder with damage of blood vessels manifested as urinary bleeding, frequent, urgent, painful, and difficult dark urine with a burning sensation, red tongue with thin yellow coat, a rapid pulse.

■ Cautions and Contraindications
It is contraindicated in cases of chronic urinary bleeding with weak constitution. Use with caution for patients with deficiency of the spleen and stomach. Do not use overdose and for long term.

■ Modern Applications
Acute UTI, lithangiuria, acute glomerulonephritis, renal tuberculosis etc.
This formula can be used for patient with bloody urine seen by the naked eye or macroscopic hematuria.

376

Xiao Jian Zhong Tang-Minor Strengthen the Middle Burner Decoction

Minor Cinnamon and Peony Combination

小 建 中 汤

■ **Ingredients**

Bai Shao Yao	White Peony	18g
Gui Zhi	Cinnamon Twig	9g
Zhi Gan Cao	Baked Licorice	6g
Sheng Jiang	Fresh Ginger	9g
Da Zao	Jujube	12pcs
Yi Tang	Maltose	18-30g

■ **Preparation**

Use as decoction or prepared form.

■ **Pertaining Category**

Middle Burner Warming and Cold Dispelling

■ **Functions**

Warms and tonifies middle burner gently, dispels cold. Relieves spasmodic abdominal pain.

■ **Indications**

Chronic mild spleen Qi deficiency and deficient cold in the middle burner manifested as prolonged intermittent, spasmodic abdominal pain which can be alleviated by local warmth and pressure, pale complexion, poor appetite, or palpitation, restlessness, or lower grade fever, or mild aching and cold limbs, pale tongue with white coat, a thin, wiry, and weak pulse.

■ **Cautions and Contraindications**

It is contraindicated in cases of vomiting, round worms, abdominal distention, and heat from Yin deficiency.

■ **Modern Applications**

Gastritis, peptic ulcer, inflammatory bowel disease, chronic hepatitis chronic appendicitis, gastric and intestinal spasms, neurasthenia, aplastic anemia, postpartum fever, etc.

Xiao Ke Fang-Wasting Thirst Formula
Rehmannia and Trichosanthes Formula
消 渴 方

■ **Ingredients**

Sheng Di Huang	Dried Rehmannia	15g
Tian Hua Fen	Trichosanthes Root	15g
Huang Lian	Coptis	6g
Ou Jie(Zhi)	Lotus Node	9-20g
Feng Mi	Honey	20g
Sheng Jiang(Zhi)	Fresh Ginger	3-6g
Ren Ru Zhi	Human Milk	50ml

■ **Preparation**

Use as decoction or prepared form. "Zhi" (Juices) should be stirred into the strained decoction.

■ **Pertaining Category**

Additional Formulas for Internal Medicine

■ **Functions**

Clears heat, moistens the lungs, generates body fluids, relieves thirst.

■ Indications

Upper burner pattern of diabetes with lung heat and damage of Yin fluids manifested as excessive thirst, a strong desire to drink fluids, dry mouth, frequent urination, or hungry easily, dry tongue with red tip, sides, and thin yellow coat, a rapid pulse.

■ Cautions and Contraindications

None noted.

■ Modern Applications

Diabetes, etc.

Ren Ru Zhi (Human Milk) can be substituted by cow milk.

Xiao Qing Long Tang-Minor Bluegreen Dragon Decoction
Minor Blue Dragon Combination
小青龙汤

■ Ingredients

Ma Huang	Ephedra	9g
Gui Zhi	Cinnamon Twig	6g
Bai Shao Yao	White Peony	9g
Gan Jiang	Dried Ginger	9g
Xi Xin	Asarum	3g
Wu Wei Zi	Schisandra	3g
Ban Xia	Pinellia Tuber	9g
Zhi Gan Cao	Baked Licorice	6g

■ Preparation

Use as decoction or prepared form.

■ Pertaining Category

Pungent Warm Exterior Relieving

Functions

Promotes sweat, expels wind-cold, releases the exterior. Opens and warms the lungs, transforms phlegm-fluid, relieves coughing and wheezing.

■ Indications

Exterior wind-cold with interior phlegm-fluid retention manifested as aversion to wind-cold, fever, absence of sweating, body aches, cough, difficulty in breathing, profuse white thin sputum, no thirst or thirst with no desire to drink, or retching, or diarrhea, or edema of head, face, and limbs, white moist tongue coat, a superficial, tight pulse.

■ Cautions and Contraindications

It is contraindicated in cases of coughing of blood, dry cough, dry mouth and throat, and cough with thick yellow sputum. Do not use overdose and for long term. Use with caution for patients with hypertension and heart problems.

■ Modern Applications

Influenza, acute and chronic bronchitis, bronchial asthma, pulmonary emphysema, etc.

Xiao Xian Xiong Tang-Minor Sinking into Chest Decoction
Minor Trichosanthes Combination
小 陷 胸 汤

■ Ingredients

Huang Lian	*Coptis*	6g
Ban Xia	*Pinellia Tuber*	12g
Gua Lou	*Trichosanthes Fruit*	30g

■ Preparation

Use as decoction or prepared form.

380

- **Pertaining Category**

Heat Clearing and Phlegm Resolving

- **Functions**

Clears heat, resolves phlegm. Opens the chest, disperses clumps.

- **Indications**

Phlegm-heat accumulating in the chest and epigastrium manifested as a fullness sensation in the chest and epigastrium that is painful with pressure, cough with yellow, thick, and sticky sputum, dark and scanty urine, constipation, red tongue with yellow greasy coat, a slippery, rapid pulse.

- **Cautions and Contraindications**

It is contraindicated in cases of loose stools or diarrhea due to significant spleen and stomach deficiency.

- **Modern Applications**

Acute or chronic bronchitis, pneumonia, pleurisy, cholecystitis, acute or chronic gastritis, peptic ulcer, angina pectoris, intercostal neuralgia, etc.

Xiao Yao San-Wandering Powder
Bupleurum and Tang-kuei Combination
逍 遥 散

- **Ingredients**

Chai Hu	Bupleurum	9g
Dang Gui	Chinese Angelica	9g
Bai Shao Yao	White Peony	12g
Bai Zhu	White Atractylodes	9g
Fu Ling	Hoelen/Poria	15g
Bo He	Peppermint	3g
Wei Jiang	Roasted Ginger	6g
Zhi Gan Cao	Baked Licorice	6g

■ **Preparation**
Use as decoction or prepared form.

■ **Pertaining Category**
Regulating the Liver and Spleen (Mediating)

■ **Functions**
Disperses liver Qi, relieves stagnation. Tonifies the spleen Qi, nourishes blood, regulates menstruation.

■ **Indications**
Stagnation of the liver Qi with deficiency of the spleen Qi and blood manifested as hypochondriac distending pain, fullness in the chest and epigastrium, headache, blurred vision, dryness in the mouth and throat, lassitude, poor appetite, loose stools, irregular menstruation, breast distention, or alternate chills and fever, pale red tongue with thin white coat, a wiry, weak pulse.

■ **Cautions and Contraindications**
None noted.

■ **Modern Applications**
Chronic hepatitis, chronic gastritis, peptic ulcer, neurosis, irregular menstruation, premenstrual syndrome, menopausal syndrome, fibrocystic breasts, mental depression, hysteria, etc.

Xie Bai San-Drain the White Powder
Morus and Lycium Formula
泻 白 散

■ **Ingredients**

Di Gu Pi	*Lycium Bark*	30g
Sang Bai Pi	*Morus Bark*	30g
Zhi Gan Cao	*Baked Licorice*	3g
Geng Mi	*Oryza*	12-15g

■ **Preparation**
Use as decoction or prepared form.

■ **Pertaining Category**
Clearing Heat from Zang-fu Organs

■ **Functions**
Drains accumulated heat from lungs, relieves cough and asthma.

■ **Indications**
Heat in the lungs manifested as cough, wheezing, difficulty in breathing, feverish skin which is worse in the afternoon, red tongue with yellow coat, a thin, rapid pulse.

■ **Cautions and Contraindications**
It is contraindicated in cases of cough and asthma due to deficient cold or exterior wind-cold invasion.

■ **Modern Applications**
Asthma, bronchitis, infantile measles, pneumonia, pulmonary tuberculosis, whooping cough, etc.

Xie Huang San-Drain the Yellow Powder
Siler and Licorice Formula
泻黄散

■ **Ingredients**

Huo Xiang	Agastache	21g
Zhi Zi	Gardenia Fruit	6g
Shi Gao	Gypsum	15g
Fang Feng	Siler	120g
Gan Cao	Licorice	90g

■ **Preparation**
Use as prepared form or decoction with properly adjusted dosage.

■ Pertaining Category
Clearing Heat from Zang-fu Organs

■ Functions
Drains latent fire from the spleen and stomach.

■ Indications
Latent fire or damp-heat in the spleen and stomach manifested as mouth ulcers, foul breath, irritability, strong thirst, excessive hunger, dry mouth and lips, or unusual movement of the tongue seen in children, red and dry tongue with yellow coat, a rapid pulse.

■ Cautions and Contraindications
It is contraindicated in cases of stomach Yin and Qi deficiency.

■ Modern Applications
Recurrent aphthous ulcers, stomatitis, glossitis, etc.

Xie Xin Tang-Drain the Heart Decoction
Coptis and Rhubarb Combination
泻心汤

■ Ingredients

Huang Lian	Coptis	3g
Huang Qin	Scute	9g
Da Huang	Rhubarb	6g

■ Preparation
Use as decoction or prepared form.

■ Pertaining Category
Heat Clearing and Detoxicating

■ Functions
Drains fire-heat from heart and stomach, relieves toxicity. Drains dampness, purges stagnation. Cools blood, stops bleeding.

Indications

Toxic heat or damp-heat in the upper and middle burners manifested as vomiting of blood, nosebleeding, jaundice, irritability, a stifling sensation in the chest, red, swelling, and painful eyes, ulceration of tongue and mouth, or carbuncles and boils, constipation, red tongue with yellow greasy coat, a slippery, rapid pulse.

■ Cautions and Contraindications

It is contraindicated in cases of the spleen and stomach Yang deficiency or Yin deficiency with deep-red and uncoated tongue.

■ Modern Applications

Influenza, encephalitis B, meningitis, septicemia, pyogenic skin infection, hepatitis, acute gastroenteritis or dysentery, acute UTI, acute cholecystitis, as well as stomatitis, toothache, and laryngopharyngitis, etc.

Xin Jia Huang Long Tang-Newly Augmented Yellow Dragon Decoction
新加黄龙汤

■ Ingredients

Da Huang	Rhubarb	9g
Mang Xiao	Mirabilitum	3g
Xuan Shen	Scrophularia	15g
Sheng Di Huang	Dried Rehmannia	15g
Mai Men Dong	Ophiopogon	15g
Hai Shen	Strichopus	2pcs
Ren Shen	Ginseng	4.5g
Dang Gui	Chinese Angelica	4.5g
Gan Cao	Licorice	6g
Jiang Zhi	Ginger Juice	6 teaspoons

■ Preparation
Use as decoction or prepared form. Ren Shen should be decocted separately for 1-2 hours, then mixed with decoction of other herbs.

■ Pertaining Category
Purging Downward with Tonifying Effect

■ Functions
Nourishes Yin, tonifies Qi. Moves bowel, purges the accumulated heat downward.

■ Indications
Interior heat accumulation with deficiency of Qi, Yin, and blood manifested as constipation, abdominal distention and hardness, lassitude, shortness of breath, dry mouth and throat, chapped lips with fissures on the tongue, dry yellow or black tongue coat, a deep thin, and weak pulse.

■ Cautions and Contraindications
None noted.

■ Modern Applications
Intestinal obstruction, elderly, postpartum, or habitual constipation, epidemic or non-epidemic febrile diseases, etc.

Xin Jia Xiang Ru Yin-Newly Augmented Elsholtzia Beverage
Elsholtzia and Lonicera Combination
新加香薷饮

■ Ingredients

Xiang Ru	Elsholtzia	6g
Jin Yin Hua	Lonicera	9g
Bian Dou Hua	Dolichos	9g
Lian Qiao	Forsythia Fruit	6g
Hou Po	Magnolia Bark	6g

- **Preparation**

Use as decoction or prepared form.

- **Pertaining Category**

Summer Heat Clearing

- **Functions**

Expels summer heat and cold, relieves the exterior. Clears heat, transforms dampness.

- **Indications**

Early stage of summer heat with externally contracted wind-cold manifested as fever, headache, slight aversion to cold, absence of sweating, thirst, red face, sore throat, a stifling sensation in the chest, irritability, white greasy coat, a superficial, flooding, and rapid pulse.

- **Cautions and Contraindications**

None noted.

- **Modern Applications**

Common cold in the summer, acute laryngopharyngitis, etc.

Xing Su San-Apricot Seed and Perilla Powder

Apricot Seed and Perilla Formula

杏 苏 散

■ Ingredients

Zi Su Ye	Perilla Leaf	6g
Xing Ren	Apricot Seed	6g
Ban Xia	Pinellia Tuber	6g
Fu Ling	Hoelen/Poria	6g
Chen Pi	Tangerine Peel	6g
Qian Hu	Hogfennel Root	6g
Jie Geng	Platycodon	6g
Zhi Ke	Bitter Orange	6g
Sheng Jiang	Fresh Ginger	6g
Da Zao	Jujube	2pcs
Gan Cao	Licorice	3g

■ Preparation
Use as decoction or prepared form.

■ Pertaining Category
Moistening Dryness

■ Functions
Gently expels wind-cold and dryness, disperses the lung Qi, resolves phlegm, relieves cough.

■ Indications
External wind-cold and dryness attacking the lungs manifested as mild headache, slight aversion to cold, absence of sweating, cough with clear sputum which is not easy to expectorate, stuffy nose, dry throat, thin white tongue coat, a wiry pulse.

■ Cautions and Contraindications
It is contraindicated in cases of cough due to wind-heat, phlegm-heat, or deficient patterns.

■ Modern Applications
Common cold, bronchitis, upper respiratory infection, emphysema, etc.

388

Xiong Zhi Shi Gao Tang-Ligusticum, Angelica Root, and Gypsum Decoction
Ligusticum and Angelica Root Combination
芎芷石膏汤

■ **Ingredients**

Chuan Xiong	Ligusticum	6g
Bai Zhi	Angelica Root	6g
Shi Gao	Gypsum	18g
Ju Hua	Chrysanthemum	9g
Gao Ben	Straw Weed	6g
Qiang Huo	Notopterygium	6g

■ **Preparation**
Use as decoction or prepared form.

■ **Pertaining Category**
External Wind Expelling

■ **Functions**
Expels wind-heat, alleviates pain.

■ **Indications**
External wind-heat attacking the collaterals on the head manifested as sudden severe distending headache, or facial pain, or toothache, fever, aversion to wind, red complexion and eyes, thirst with a desire to drink cold water, dark and scanty urine, constipation, red tongue with yellow coat, a superficial, rapid pulse.

■ **Cautions and Contraindications**
It is contraindicated for headache due to wind-cold invasion or deficiency.

■ **Modern Applications**
Headache, sinus, toothache, trigeminal nueralgia, etc.

Xuan Fu Dai Zhe Tang-Elecampane Flower and Hematite Decoction
Inula and Hematite Combination
旋复代赭汤

■ **Ingredients**

Xuan Fu Hua	Elecampane Flower	9g
Dai Zhe Shi	Hematite	9-15g
Ren Shen	Ginseng	6g
Ban Xia	Pinellia Tuber	9g
Sheng Jiang	Fresh Ginger	6-9g
Da Zao	Jujube	4pcs
Zhi Gan Cao	Baked Licorice	3-6g

■ **Preparation**
Use as decoction or prepared form. Xuan Fu Hua should be wrapped in gauze when making decoction. Dai Zhe Shi may be decocted first for 20 minutes.

■ **Pertaining Category**
Qi Regulating(Descending)

■ **Functions**
Descends the rebellious Qi, resolves phlegm. Tonifies Qi, harmonizes the stomach.

■ **Indications**
Turbid-phlegm accumulation with deficient and rebellious stomach Qi manifested as epigastric fullness and rigidity, frequent belching, sour regurgitation, vomiting, salivation, or cough and wheezing, pale tongue with white moist coat, a wiry, weak pulse.

■ Cautions and Contraindications

None noted.

■ Modern Applications

Chronic gastritis, peptic ulcer, gastric neurosis, neurogenic hiccups or vomiting, Meniere's syndrome, incomplete pyloric obstruction, etc.

Xue Fu Zhu Yu Tang-Remove Stasis from the Mansion of Blood Decoction

Decoction for Removing Blood Stasis in the Chest

血府逐瘀汤

■ Ingredients

Tao Ren	Peach Kernel	12g
Hong Hua	Safflower	9g
Dang Gui	Chinese Angelica	9g
Sheng Di Huang	Dried Rehmannia	9g
Chuan Xiong	Ligusticum	5g
Chi Shao Yao	Red Peony	6g
Chuan Niu Xi	Cyathula	9g
Jie Geng	Platycodon	5g
Chai Hu	Bupleurum	3g
Zhi Ke	Bitter Orange	6g
Gan Cao	Licorice	3g

■ Preparation

Use as decoction or prepared form.

■ Pertaining Category

Blood Invigorating

■ Functions

Promotes the circulation of blood and Qi, removes blood stasis, relieves pain.

■ **Indications**

Blood stasis in the chest with liver qi stagnation manifested as prolonged chest pain or headache marked by piercing and fixed in location, or chronic hiccups, dry heaves, and choking when drinking water, palpitation, insomnia, irritability, easily to get angry, or increased body temperature in the evening, purplish lips, darkness around eyes, dark red or purple tongue, a hesitant, wiry, or tight pulse.

■ **Cautions and Contraindications**

It is contraindicated during pregnancy and in cases of excessive menstrual bleeding, bleeding diathesis, any bleeding disorders, etc.

■ **Modern Applications**

Coronary artery disease, rheumatic valvular heart disease, cerebral vascular accident, trigeminal neuralgia, intercostal neuralgia, cirrhosis of liver, splenomegaly, dysmenorrhea, headache due to trauma, etc.

Yan Hu Suo San-Corydalis Powder
Corydalis Formula
延胡索散

■ **Ingredients**

Yan Hu Suo	*Corydalis*	15g
Dang Gui	*Chinese Angelica*	15g
Chi Shao Yao	*Red Peony*	15g
Pu Huang	*Cattail Pollen*	15g
Rou Gui	*Cinnamon Bark*	15g
Jiang Huang	*Tumeric Rhizome*	9g
Ru Xiang	*Frankincense*	9g
Mo Yao	*Myrrh*	9g
Mu Xiang	*Saussurea*	9g
Zhi Gan Cao	*Baked Licorice*	7g
Sheng Jiang	*Fresh Ginger*	7slices

■ **Preparation**

Use as decoction or prepared form.

■ **Pertaining Category**

Qi Regulating(Moving)

■ **Functions**

Moves Qi, promotes blood circulation. Regulates menses. Dispels cold, stops pain.

■ **Indications**

Stagnation of blood and Qi due to cold or emotional stress manifested as epigastric and abdominal pain referring to hypochondrium or lumbar areas, severe menstrual cramps, irregular menstruation with dark colored blood or clots, purple tongue or purplish spots on the tongue, a wiry, hesitant pulse.

■ **Cautions and Contraindications**

It is contraindicated during pregnancy.

■ **Modern Applications**

Dysmenorrhea, irregular menstruation, endometriosis, gastritis, etc

Yang He Tang-Yang Harmony Decoction
Yang Heartening Decoction
阳和汤

■ **Ingredients**

Shu Di Huang	Cooked Rehmannia	30g
Rou Gui	Cinnamon Bark	3g
Lu Jiao Jiao	Colloid of Antler	9g
Bai Jie Zi	Brassica Seed	6g
Jiang Tan	Baked Ginger	2g
Ma Huang	Ephedra	2g
Gan Cao	Licorice	3g

■ Preparation
Use as decoction or prepared form.

■ Pertaining Category
Treating External Carbuncles

■ Functions
Warms Yang, nourishes blood. Expels cold, resolves phlegm, clears obstruction.

■ Indications
Carbuncles due to cold-phlegm obstruction with Yang and blood deficiency manifested as spreaded swelling of affected area without purulent core and color change of skin, localized pain without warmth, slow progression, absence of fever and thirst, or swollen joints with atrophy, pale tongue with white coat, a deep, weak, and thin pulse.

■ Cautions and Contraindications
It is contraindicated in cases of carbuncles with excess heat or Yin deficiency with deficient heat. Use with extreme caution for patients with hypertension and heart problems.

■ Modern Applications
Bone tuberculosis, lymphoid tuberculosis, thromboangiitis obliterans chronic osteomyelitis, carbuncle of Yin type, chronic deep-rooted abscess, etc.

Yang Jing Zhong Yu Tang-Nourish Essence and Plant Jade Decoction
养精种玉汤

■ Ingredients

Dang Gui	Chinese Angelica	12g
Bai Shao Yao	White Peony	12g
Shu Di Huang	Cooked Rehmannia	24g
Shan Zhu Yu	Dogwood Fruit	12g

■ Preparation
Use as decoction or prepared form.

■ Pertaining Category
Additional Formulas for Ob-Gyn Disorders

■ Functions
Nourishes Yin and blood, benefits essence. Regulates Chong and Ren channels.

■ Indications
Infertility due to kidney Yin and essence deficiency manifested as inability to conceive, antedated or normal menstrual cycles, scanty and red colored menses without blood clots, soreness and weakness of lower back, emaciation, dizziness, blurred vision, palpitation, insomnia, dry mouth, five hearts heat, lower fever in the afternoon, light red tongue with scanty coat, a thin rapid pulse.

■ Cautions and Contraindications
None noted.

■ Modern Applications
Infertility, amenorrhea, anemia, neurasthenia, etc.
For best result, add Han Lian Cao(Eclipta)12g, Nu Zhen Zi(Ligustrum)12g.

Yang Xin Tang-Nourish the Heart Decoction
Astragalus and Zizyphus Combination
养心汤

■ Ingredients

Sheng Di Huang	Dried Rehmannia	9g
Shu Di Huang	Cooked Rehmannia	9g
Dang Gui	Chinese Angelica	9g
Ren Shen	Ginseng	12g
Mai Men Dong	Ophiopogon	12g
Suan Zao Ren	Zizyphus	12g
Fu Shen	Hoelen/Poria	9g
Bai Zi Ren	Biota Seed	6g
Wu Wei Zi	Schisandra Fruit	6g
Zhi Gan Cao	Baked Licorice	3g
Lian Zi	Lotus Seed	6g
Deng Xin Cao	Rush Pith	6g

■ Preparation

Use as decoction or prepared form.

■ Pertaining Category

Spirit Calming with Nourishing Sedative Herbs

■ Functions

Tonifies the heart Qi, nourishes the heart blood and Yin, calms spirit.

■ Indications

Heart Qi, blood, and Yin deficiency manifested as palpitation, restlessness, insomnia, anxiety, poor memory, pale tongue with thin white coat, a thin, weak pulse.

■ Cautions and Contraindications

None noted.

■ Modern Applications

Neurasthenia, chronic heart diseases, insomnia, cardiac neurosis, etc.

This formula is from "Gu Jin Yi Tong Da Quan"(Comprehensive Collection of Medicine Past and Present).

Yang Yin Qing Fei Tang-Nourish Yin and Clear the Lung Decoction

Rehmannia and Fritillary Combination
养 阴 清 肺 汤

■ Ingredients

Sheng Di Huang	Dried Rehmannia	6g
Mai Men Dong	Ophiopogon	5g
Xuan Shen	Scrophularia	5g
Chuan Bei Mu	Tendrilled Fritillary	3g
Mu Dan Pi	Moutan Bark	3g
Bai Shao Yao	White Peony	3g
Bo He	Peppermint	2g
Gan Cao	Licorice	2g

■ Preparation
Use as decoction or prepared form.

■ Pertaining Category
Moistening Dryness

■ Functions
Nourishes Yin, clears lung heat, benefits throat.

■ Indications
Diphtheria with lung Yin deficiency manifested as fever, dry nasal cavity and lips, or dry hacking cough, difficulty in breathing, sore throat with white membrane in the throat, which is hard to be removed, hoarse voice, red and dry tongue, a weak, thin, and rapid pulse.

■ Cautions and Contraindications
Extreme attention should be paid when treating this serious or even life-threatening disease(diphtheria); western medicine should be used as combination, especially in case of difficult breathing.

■ Modern Applications
Diphtheria, acute pharyngitis, acute tonsillitis, etc.

Yi Guan Jian-Linking Brew
Glehnia and Rehmannia Combination
一贯煎

■ **Ingredients**

Sha Shen	*Glehnia Root*	10g
Mai Men Dong	*Ophiopogon*	10g
Dang Gui	*Chinese Angelica*	10g
Sheng Di Huang	*Dried Rehmannia*	30g
Gou Qi Zi	*Lycium Fruit*	12g
Chuan Lian Zi	*Melia*	5g

■ **Preparation**
Use as decoction or prepared form.

■ **Pertaining Category**
Yin Tonifying

■ **Functions**
Nourishes the liver and kidney Yin. Soothes the liver, relieves Qi stagnation.

■ **Indications**
Yin deficiency of the liver and kidney with liver Qi stagnation manifested as distending pain in the thoracic, hypochondriac, and epigastric regions, fullness in the chest, sore regurgitation, a bitter taste in the mouth, dry mouth and throat, or abdominal mass, or hernial pain, red and dry tongue with scanty coat, a thin, weak, wiry or rapid pulse.

■ **Cautions and Contraindications**
It is contraindicated in cases of phlegm-dampness retention.

■ **Modern Applications**
Chronic hepatitis, early stage of liver cirrhosis, chronic gastritis, peptic ulcer, diabetes, hypertension, etc.

Yi Huang Tang-Change Yellow(Discharge) Decoction
易 黄 汤

■ **Ingredients**

Shan Yao	Dioscorea	30g
Huang Bai	Phellodendron	6g
Qian Shi	Euryale Seed	30g
Bai Guo	Ginkgo Nut	10pcs
Che Qian Zi	Plantago Seed	3g

■ **Preparation**
Use as decoction or prepared form. Che Qian Zi should be wrapped in gauze when making decoction.

■ **Pertaining Category**
Stabilizing the Menses and Stopping Leukorrhea

■ **Functions**
Tonifies the spleen, dries dampness. Clears heat, stops leukorrhea.

■ **Indications**
Damp-heat in the lower burner with mild spleen Qi deficiency manifested as yellow or white, thick vaginal discharge with a bad fishy smell, heaviness in the limbs, reduced appetite, thin greasy yellow or white tongue coat, a slippery, or weak pulse.

■ **Cautions and Contraindications**
This formula should be used in moderate damp-heat condition. It should not be used in cases without damp-heat or with severe damp-heat.

■ **Modern Applications**
Leukorrhea, inflammation of the genital system, vaginitis, cervicitis, etc.

Yi Wei Tang-Benefit the Stomach Decoction
Glehnia and Ophiopogon Combination
益 胃 汤

■　　**Ingredients**

Sha Shen	Glehnia Root	9g
Mai Men Dong	Ophiopogon	15g
Sheng Di Huang	Dried Rehmannia	15g
Yu Zhu	Polygonatum	4.5g
Bing Tang	Rock Candy	3g

■　　**Preparation**
Use as decoction or prepared form.

■　　**Pertaining Category**
Yin Tonifying

■　　**Functions**
Nourishes the stomach Yin, generates body fluids, moistens dryness.

■　　**Indications**
Yin deficiency of the stomach manifested as dry mouth and throat, thirst, increased appetite, or bleeding gums, slight red and dry tongue with scanty coat, a thin pulse.

■　　**Cautions and Contraindications**
It is contraindicated in cases of poor appetite and diarrhea due to deficiency of the spleen and stomach.

■　　**Modern Applications**
Chronic gastritis, gingivitis, later stage of febrile diseases, diabetes, etc.

Yi Yi Fu Zi Bai Jiang San-Coix, Aconite, and Baijiang Powder

Coicis, Prepared Aconite, and Patrinia Powder
薏苡附子敗醬散

■ **Ingredients**

Yi Yi Ren	*Coix Seed*	24-30g
Shu Fu Zi	*Prepared Aconite*	6-9g
Bai Jiang Cao	*Patrinia*	15-18g

■ **Preparation**
Use as decoction or prepared form.

■ **Pertaining Category**
Treating Internal Abscess

■ **Functions**
Promotes pus discharge, reduces swelling.

■ **Indications**
Intestinal abscess with formation of pus due to damp-cold and stagnant blood manifested as tightness and distention in the right lower abdomen that feels soft when palpating, dry and squamous skin, absence of fever, a rapid pulse.

■ **Cautions and Contraindications**
It is contraindicated for early stage of intestinal abscess due to damp-heat and without formation of pus.

■ **Modern Applications**
Chronic appendicitis with formation of pus and is not suitable for purgation.

Yi Yi Ren Tang-Coix Seed Decoction
Coix Seed Combination
薏苡仁汤

■ **Ingredients**

Yi Yi Ren	Coix Seed	9g
Mu Dan Pi	Moutan Bark	6g
Tao Ren	Peach Kernel	6g
Gua Lou Ren	Trichosanthes Seed	9g

■ **Preparation**
Use as decoction or prepared form.

■ **Pertaining Category**
Treating Internal Abscess

■ **Functions**
Drains dampness, moistens the intestines. Promotes blood circulation, stops pain.

■ **Indications**
Early stage of intestinal abscess with dampness retention and stagnant blood manifested as colicky pain in the lower abdomen with distention, poor appetite, difficult urination, or postpartum abdominal pain, abdominal pain before or after menstruation, purple tongue with greasy coat, a wiry, hesitant pulse.

■ **Cautions and Contraindications**
It is contraindicated during pregnancy.

■ **Modern Applications**
Chronic appendicitis without complication, purulent appendicitis, acute annexitis, pelvic inflammatory disease, lochioschesis, etc.
This formula is from "Zheng Zhi Zhun Sheng "(Standards of Patterns and Treatments).

Yin Chen Hao Tang-Capillaris Decoction
Capillaris Combination
茵 陈 蒿 汤

■ **Ingredients**

Yin Chen Hao	*Oriental Wormwood*	18g
Zhi Zi	*Gardenia Fruit*	9g
Da Huang	*Rhubarb*	6g

■ **Preparation**
Use as decoction or prepared form.

■ **Pertaining Category**
Damp-heat Clearing

■ **Functions**
Clears heat, drains dampness, eliminates jaundice.

■ **Indications**
Yang jaundice due to damp-heat manifested as bright orange-yellow coloration of skin and eyes, slight abdominal distention, thirst, difficult and dark urination, red tongue with yellow greasy coat, a deep, slippery, and rapid pulse.

■ **Cautions and Contraindications**
It is contraindicated for patients with Yin jaundice due to damp-cold.

■ **Modern Applications**
Acute infectious icteric hepatitis, acute pancreatitis, cholecystitis, cholelithiasis, etc.

Yin Chen Wu Ling San-Five Ingredients Powder with Poria plus Capillaris
Capillaris and Hoelen Five Formula
茵 陈 五 苓 散

■ **Ingredients**

Yin Chen Hao	Oriental Wormwood	15-30g
Fu Ling	Hoelen/Poria	9g
Zhu Ling	Polyporus	9g
Bai Zhu	White Atractylodes	9g
Ze Xie	Alisma Tuber	12g
Gui Zhi	Cinnamon Twig	6g

■ **Preparation**
Use as decoction or prepared form.

■ **Pertaining Category**
Downward Dampness Draining

■ **Functions**
Promotes urination, drains dampness. Purges heat, reduces jaundice

■ **Indications**
Yang jaundice due to damp-heat with pronounced dampness manifested as slight orange-yellow coloration of skin and eyes, abdominal distention, difficult urination, white or yellow greasy tongue coat, a deep, slippery pulse.

■ **Cautions and Contraindications**
None noted.

■ **Modern Applications**
Acute infectious icteric hepatitis, acute pancreatitis, cholecystitis, cholelithiasis, etc.

Yin Chen Zhu Fu Tang-Oriental Wormwood, Atractylodes, and Aconite Decoction
Capillaris, Atractylodes, and Aconite Combination
茵 陈 术 附 汤

■ Ingredients

Yin Chen Hao	Oriental Wormwood	12g
Bai Zhu	White Atractylodes	9g
Zhi Fu Zi	Prepared Aconite	6g
Gan Jiang	Dried Ginger	9g
Rou Gui	Cinnamon Bark	3g
Zhi Gan Cao	Baked Licorice	6g

■ Preparation
Use as decoction or prepared form.

■ Pertaining Category
Additional Formulas for Internal Medicine

■ Functions
Strengthens the spleen, harmonizes the stomach. Warms and transforms cold-dampness.

■ Indications
Yin jaundice due to damp-cold and spleen Yang deficiency manifested as dull smoky yellow discoloration of the eyes and skin poor appetite, epigastric fullness and abdominal distention, loose stools, listlessness, aversion to cold, cold limbs, absence of thirst, pale tongue with white greasy coat, a soft, slow, and deep pulse.

■ Cautions and Contraindications
It is contraindicated in cases of jaundice due to damp-heat.

■ Modern Applications
Chronic hepatitis, liver cirrhosis, hepatic necrosis, etc.

Yin Qiao San-Lonicera Flower and Forsythia Powder
Lonicera and Forsythia Formula
银 翘 散

■ Ingredients

Jin Yin Hua	*Lonicera*	9g
Lian Qiao	*Forsythia Fruit*	9g
Jie Geng	*Platycodon*	6g
Bo He	*Peppermint*	6g
Zhu Ye	*Bamboo Leaf*	4g
Gan Cao	*Licorice*	5g
Jing Jie Sui	*Schizonepeta Spike*	5g
Dan Dou Chi	*Prepared Soybean*	5g
Niu Bang Zi	*Burdock Fruit*	9g
Lu Gen	*Reed Rhizome*	6g

■ Preparation
Use as decoction or prepared form. Do not cook for more than 20 minutes. Bo He should be added 5 minutes near the end of cooking.

■ Pertaining Category
Pungent Cool Exterior Relieving

■ Functions
Expels wind-heat, releases the exterior. Clears internal heat, relieves toxicity, benefits throat.

■ Indications
Invasion of wind-heat or early stage of epidemic febrile disease manifested as fever, slight aversion to wind-cold, absence of sweating or with little sweating, throbbing headache, severe sore throat and thirst, red tip tongue with thin white or thin yellow coat, a superficial, rapid pulse.

■ Cautions and Contraindications
It is contraindicated in cases of wind-cold invasion.

■ Modern Applications
Common cold, influenza, acute tonsillitis, acute laryngopharyngitis, early stage of measles and parotitis, urticaria, epidemic encephalitis B, early stage of pneumonia or lung abscess, etc.

You Gui Wan-Right Restoring Pill
Restore Right Pill
右归丸

■ **Ingredients**

Shu Di Huang	Cooked Rehmannia	240g
Shan Zhu Yu	Dogwood Fruit	90g
Shan Yao	Dioscorea	120g
Gou Qi Zi	Lycium Fruit	120g
Tu Si Zi	Dodder Seed	120g
Lu Jiao Jiao	Colloid of Antler	120g
Du Zhong	Eucommia Bark	120g
Dang Gui	Chinese Angelica	90g
Rou Gui	Cinnamon Bark	60-120g
Fu Zi	Prepared Aconite	60-180g

■ **Preparation**
Use as prepared form.

■ **Pertaining Category**
Yang Tonifying

■ **Functions**
Warms the kidney yang, tonifies the kidney Qi. Nourishes essence and blood.

■ **Indications**
Deficiency of the kidney Yang and essence with decline of Mingmen fire and blood deficiency manifested as listlessness, aversion to cold, cold limbs, impotence, seminal emission, infertility, or diarrhea with undigested food, frequent urination or incontinence, soreness and weakness of lower back and knees, or edema, pale tongue with thin white coat, a deep, weak, and slow pulse.

■ **Cautions and Contraindications**
It is contraindicated in cases of deficient fire due to Yin deficiency.

■ **Modern Applications**
Chronic nephritis, diabetes, impotence, spermatorrhea, neurasthenia, menopausal syndrome, optic nerve atrophy, etc.

You Gui Yin-Right Restoring Beverage
Restore Right Beverage
右 归 饮

■ **Ingredients**

Shu Di Huang	Cooked Rehmannia	6-30g
Shan Zhu Yu	Dogwood Fruit	3g
Shan Yao	Dioscorea	6g
Gou Qi Zi	Lycium Fruit	6g
Du Zhong	Eucommia Bark	6g
Rou Gui	Cinnamon Bark	6g
Fu Zi	Prepared Aconite	9g
Zhi Gan Cao	Baked Licorice	6g

■ **Preparation**
Use as decoction or prepared form.

■ **Pertaining Category**
Yang Tonifying

■ **Functions**
Warms the kidney Yang. Supplements the kidney essence.

■ **Indications**
Mild deficiency of the kidney Yang and essence manifested as soreness in the lower back, abdominal pain, cold limbs, listlessness, lassitude, frequent, clear urine, impotence, pale tongue with thin white coat, a deep, thin, and weak pulse; as well as flushed face due to true cold with false heat.

408

■ Cautions and Contraindications
It is contraindicated in cases of deficiency fire due to Yin deficiency.

■ Modern Applications
Chronic nephritis, diabetes, impotence, spermatorrhea, neurasthenia, menopausal syndrome, optic nerve atrophy, etc.

Yu Nu Jian-Jade Woman Brew
Rehmannia and Gypsum Combination
玉女煎

■ Ingredients

Shi Gao	Gypsum	15-30g
Shu Di Huang	Cooked Rehmannia	9-30g
Mai Men Dong	Ophiopogon	6-9g
Zhi Mu	Anemarrhena	4.5g
Niu Xi	Achyranthes	4.5g

■ Preparation
Use as decoction or prepared form.

■ Pertaining Category
Clearing Heat from Zang-fu Organs

■ Functions
Clears heat in the stomach, nourishes Yin.

■ Indications
Stomach heat with damaged stomach Yin manifested as toothache with loosing and moving teeth, bleeding gums, frontal headache, irritability, dry mouth, thirst, or hungry easily, or diabetes condition red and dry tongue with yellow dry coat, a thin, rapid, and weak pulse.

■ Cautions and Contraindications
It is contraindicated in cases of diarrhea due to spleen and stomach deficiency.

■ Modern Applications
Periodontitis, stomatitis, glossitis, purulent swelling of gums, laryngopharyngitis, purpura, chronic gastritis, gingivitis, toothache diabetes, etc.

Yu Ping Feng San-Jade Screen Powder
玉 屏 风 散

■ Ingredients

Fang Feng	Siler	30g
Huang Qi	Astragalus	30g
Bai Zhu	White Atractylodes	60g

■ Preparation
Use as prepared form or decoction with properly reduced dosage.

■ Pertaining Category
Consolidating Exterior to Stop Sweating

■ Functions
Tonifies Qi, consolidates the superficial defense, stops sweating.

Indications

Deficiency of defensive Qi manifested as spontaneous or excessive sweating, aversion to wind, easy to catch cold or get wind rash, pale complexion, pale tongue with white coat, a superficial, weak, and soft pulse.

■ Cautions and Contraindications

It is contraindicated in cases of night sweats due to Yin deficiency and sweating caused by exterior patterns.

■ Modern Applications

Chronic rhinitis, allergic rhinitis, hyperhidrosis, person with susceptibility to the common cold, urticaria, etc.

Yu Zhen San-Jade Truth Powder
Arisaema and Typhonium Combination
玉真散

■ Ingredients

Tian Nan Xing	*Arisaema Tuber*	10g
Bai Fu Zi	*Typhonium*	10g
Qiang Huo	*Notopterygium*	10g
Tian Ma	*Gastrodia*	10g
Fang Feng	*Siler*	10g
Bai Zhi	*Angelica Root*	10g

■ Preparation

Use as powder and taken with warm water; use as decoction; or apply topically to the affected area.

■ Pertaining Category

External Wind Expelling

■ Functions

Expels wind, resolves phlegm. Relieves spasms, stops pain.

■ Indications

Tetanus due to wind and toxin invasion through a open wound manifested as lockjaw, closed mouth, stiff neck, spasms of the extremities, rigidity of the entire body, or even opisthotonos, deviated and stiff tongue, a wiry, tight pulse.

■ Cautions and Contraindications

This formula contains some toxic ingredients. It should not exceed the dosage or used long term. It is contraindicated during pregnancy.

■ Modern Applications

Tetanus, botulism, and post-traumatic pain, etc.

Yue Bi Tang-Maidservant from Yue Decoction
Ma Huang and Gypsum Combination
越婢汤

■ Ingredients

Ma Huang	Ephedra	9g
Shi Gao	Gypsum	18g
Sheng Jiang	Fresh Ginger	9g
Gan Cao	Licorice	5g
Da Zao	Jujube	5pcs

■ Preparation

Use as decoction or prepared form.

■ Pertaining Category

Pungent Cool Exterior Relieving

■ Functions

Promotes sweat, disperses the lung Qi. Induces diuresis, reduces edema.

412

Indications

Initial stage of wind edema manifested as generalized body edema that begins in the face, aversion to wind, possible slight fever, scanty urination, no thirst, thin white coat, a superficial pulse.

Cautions and Contraindications

Use cautiously for patients with hypertension and heart problems, or weak constitution.

Modern Applications

Initial stage of nephritis, edema, etc.

Yue Hua Wan-Moon Magnificence Pill
Moonlight Pill
月 华 丸

Ingredients

Tian Men Dong	*Asparagus*	30g
Mai Men Dong	*Ophiopogon*	30g
Sheng Di Huang	*Dried Rehmannia*	30g
Shu Di Huang	*Cooked Rehmannia*	30g
Shan Yao	*Dioscorea*	30g
Bai Bu	*Stemona Root*	30g
Sha Shen	*Glehnia*	30g
Chuan Bei Mu	*Tendrilled Fritillary*	30g
E Jiao	*Equus/Gelatin*	30g
Fu Ling	*Hoelen/Poria*	15g
San Qi	*Notoginseng*	15g
Ta Gan	*Lutra*	15g
Ju Hua	*Chrysanthemum*	60g
Sang Ye	*Mulberry Leaf*	60g

■ Preparation

Use as prepared form or decoction with properly reduced dosage. E Jiao should be dissolved separately in boiling water, and added into the strained decoction.

■ Pertaining Category

Yin Tonifying

■ Functions

Nourishes the lung and kidney Yin, moistens the lungs. Stops coughing and bleeding.

■ Indications

Severe Yin deficiency of the lung and kidney with dry heat in the lungs manifested as chronic or consumptive dry cough, or cough with blood tinged sputum, tidal fever, five hearts irritable heat, emaciation, dry mouth and throat, reduced appetite, a fullness sensation in the chest, shortness of breath, difficult bowel movement, dark and scanty urine, red tongue with thin yellow or no coat, a thin, weak, and rapid pulse.

■ Cautions and Contraindications

None noted.

■ Modern Applications

Middle or later stage of pulmonary tuberculosis, etc.

Yue Ju Wan-Escape Restraint Pill
Relieve Stagnancy Pill
越 鞠 丸

■ Ingredients

Xiang Fu	Cyperus Tuber	10-15g
Cang Zhu	Atractylodes	10-15g
Chuan Xiong	Ligusticum	10-15g
Shen Qu	Medicated Leaven	10-15g
Zhi Zi	Gardenia Fruit	10-15g

■ Preparation
Use as prepared form or decoction.

■ Pertaining Category
Qi Regulating(Moving)

■ Functions
Moves Qi and blood circulation, dries dampness, promotes digestion relieves stagnancy. *Formula for "6 stagnations"* — *Qi* — *Blood* — *Damp* — *Phlegm* — *Food* — *Fire*

■ Indications
Interior stagnancy from restrained liver Qi manifested as a fullness sensation in the chest, hyperchondrium, and epigastrium, abdominal distention, belching, nausea or vomiting, sour regurgitation, reduced appetite and indigestion, or cough with copious sputum, white greasy tongue coat, a wiry, slippery pulse.

■ Cautions and Contraindications
This formula is used for mild stagnation due to excess. It should not be used for stagnation caused by deficiency unless modified.

■ Modern Applications
Chronic gastritis, indigestion, peptic ulcer, gastrointestinal neurosis, cholecystitis, costal neuralgia, dysmenorrhea, etc.

Zai Zao San-Renewal Powder
Ginseng and Cinnamon Formula
再造散

- **Ingredients**

Huang Qi	Astraglus	6g
Ren Shen	Ginseng	3g
Gui Zhi	Cinnamon Twig	3g
Bai Shao Yao	Bai Shao Yao	3g
Shu Fu Zi	Prepared Aconite	3g
Xi Xin	Asarum	2g
Qiang Huo	Notopterygium	3g
Fang Feng	Siler	3g
Chuan Xiong	Ligusticum	3g
Wei Sheng Jiang	Roasted Ginger	3g
Da Zao	Jujube	2pcs
Gan Cao	Licorice	1.5g

- **Preparation**
Use as decoction or prepared form.

- **Pertaining Category**
Strengthening Body Resistance and Relieving Exterior

- **Functions**
Tonifies Qi and Yang. Promotes sweat, expels wind-cold, releases the exterior.

- **Indications**
Invasion of wind-cold with Qi and Yang deficiency constitution manifested as severe aversion to wind-cold, slight fever, lack of sweating or absence of sweating, cold limbs, lassitude, lethargy, pale complexion, weak voice, pale tongue with white coat, a deep, weak, or superficial, weak pulse.

- **Cautions and Contraindications**
Do not use this formula for patients with strong constitution. Avoid using overdose and for long term.

- **Modern Applications**
Common cold, chronic rheumatic arthritis, etc.

Zeng Ye Cheng Qi Tang-Increase the Fluids and Purge Down Digestive Qi Decoction
Rehmannia and Rhubarb Combination
增液承气汤

■ **Ingredients**

Xuan Shen	Scrophularia	30g
Mai Men Dong	Ophiopogon	25g
Sheng Di Huang	Dried Rehmannia	25g
Da Huang	Rhubarb	9g
Mang Xiao	Mirabilitum	5g

■ **Preparation**
Use as decoction or prepared form.

■ **Pertaining Category**
Purging Downward with Tonifying Effect

■ **Functions**
Nourishes Yin, generates fluids. Purges heat, promotes bowel movement.

■ **Indications**
Interior heat accumulation with Yin deficiency manifested as constipation with dry stools, dry mouth, red and dry tongue with yellow dry coat, a thin, rapid pulse.

■ **Cautions and Contraindications**
It is contraindicated during pregnancy.

■ **Modern Applications**
Habitual constipation, hemorrhoids, late stage of febrile diseases with constipation, etc.

Zeng Ye Tang-Increase the Fluids Decoction
Scrophularia and Ophiopogon Combination
增液汤

■ **Ingredients**

Xuan Shen	*Scrophularia*	30g
Mai Men Dong	*Ophiopogon*	24g
Sheng Di Huang	*Dried Rehmannia*	24g

■ **Preparation**

Use as decoction or prepared form.

■ **Pertaining Category**

Moistening Dryness

■ **Functions**

Nourishes Yin, clears heat. Moistens dryness, promotes bowel movement.

■ **Indications**

Yin deficiency with dry-heat in the Yangming system manifested as constipation, thirst, dry mouth and throat, red and dry tongue with scanty yellow coat, a deep, weak, thin, and rapid pulse.

■ **Cautions and Contraindications**

None noted.

■ **Modern Applications**

Habitual constipation, hemorrhoids, irritable bowel syndrome, hyperthyroidism, chronic pancreatitis, etc.

Zhen Gan Xi Feng Tang-Sedate the Liver and Extinguish Wind Decoction
Dragon Bone and Two Shells Combination

镇肝熄风汤

■ **Ingredients**

Niu Xi	Achyranthes Root	30g
Dai Zhe Shi	Hematite	30g
Long Gu	Dragon Bone	15g
Mu Li	Oyster Shell	15g
Gui Ban	Tortoise Plastron	15g
Bai Shao Yao	White Peony	15g
Xuan Shen	Scrophularia Root	15g
Tian Men Dong	Asparagus	15g
Chuan Lian Zi	Melia	6g
Mai Ya	Barley Sprout	6g
Yin Chen Hao	Oriental Wormwood	6g
Gan Cao	Licorice	4.5g

■ **Preparation**
Use as decoction or prepared form.

■ **Pertaining Category**
Internal Wind Extinguishing

■ **Functions**
Sedates the liver, extinguishes wind. Nourishes the liver and kidney Yin, suppresses the liver Yang.

■ **Indications**
Liver wind stirred up by liver Yang raising due to liver and kidney Yin deficiency manifested as dizziness, vertigo, tinnitus, headache, distended eyes, flushed face, irritable heat in the chest, restlessness, frequent belching, or sudden falling down with deviated mouth and eyes, inability to move the limbs and loss of sensation, or coma with failing to fully recover, red or light purple tongue with yellow coat, a wiry, forceful pulse.

419

■ **Cautions and Contraindications**

Use with caution and appropriate modification for patients with weakness of the spleen and stomach.

■ **Modern Applications**

Hypertension, cerebrovascular accident, hypertensive encephalopathy, epilepsy, cerebral arteriosclerosis, dysfunction of vegetative (Autonomic) nerve, hyperthyroidism, etc.

Zhen Ren Yang Zang Tang-True Man's Visceras Nourishing Decoction
Ginseng and Nutmeg Combination
真人养脏汤

■ **Ingredients**

Ren Shen	Ginseng	6g
Dang Gui	Chinese Angelica	9g
Bai Zhu	White Atractylodes	12g
Rou Dou Kou	Nutmeg	12g
Rou Gui	Cinnamon Bark	3g
Bai Shao Yao	White Peony	15g
Mu Xiang	Saussurea	9g
He Zi	Myrobalan Fruit	12g
Ying Su Ke	Papaver	20g
Zhi Gan Cao	Baked Licorice	6g

■ **Preparation**

Use as decoction or prepared form.

■ **Pertaining Category**

Astringing the Intestines to Stop Diarrhea

■ **Functions**

Warms and tonifies the spleen and kidney Yang, astringes the intestines, stops diarrhea.

420

Indications

Severe Yang deficiency of the spleen and kidney manifested as prolonged diarrhea or dysentery, or even incontinence of the feces, prolapse of anus, abdominal pain which is alleviated by warmth and pressure, listlessness, lassitude, soreness of lower back, cold limbs, reduced appetite, pale tongue with white coat, a deep, weak, and slow pulse.

Cautions and Contraindications

It is contraindicated for initial stage of dysentery or diarrhea with interior toxic heat.

Modern Applications

Chronic colitis, chronic dysentery, chronic enteritis, intestinal tuberculosis, prolapse of rectum, etc.

Zhen Wu Tang-True Warrior Decoction
Vitality Combination
真 武 汤

Ingredients

Fu Zi	Prepared Aconite	9g
Bai Zhu	White Atractylodes	6g
Fu Ling	Hoelen/Poria	9g
Bai Shao Yao	White Peony	9g
Sheng Jiang	Fresh Ginger	9g

Preparation

Use as decoction or prepared form.

Pertaining Category

Yang Warming and Dampness Transforming

Functions

Warms the spleen and kidney Yang, promotes urination, relieves water retention.

■ Indications

Water retention with Yang deficiency of the heart, spleen, and kidney manifested as edema, difficult urination, heaviness and pain of the limbs, abdominal pain and diarrhea, absence of thirst, or palpitation, dizziness, vomiting, pale and swollen tongue with white coat, a deep, weak, pulse.

■ Cautions and Contraindications

None noted.

■ Modern Applications

Cardiac edema, chronic nephritis, nephrotic syndrome, alimentary edema, chronic pulmonary heart disease, hypothyroidium, hypopituitarism, rheumatic heart disease, chronic gastroenteritis, liver cirrhosis, Meniere's syndrome, etc.

Zhen Zhu Mu Wan-Mother of Pearl Shell Pill
Mother of Pearl Shell Combination
珍珠母丸

■ Ingredients

Zhen Zhu Mu	Mother of Pearl	22.5g
Dang Gui	Chinese Angelica	45g
Shu Di Huang	Cooked Rehmannia	45g
Ren Shen	Ginseng	30g
Suan Zao Ren	Zizyphus	30g
Bai Zi Ren	Biota Seed	30g
Xi Jiao	Rhinoceros Horn	15g
Fu Shen	Hoelen/Poria	15g
Chen Xiang	Aquilaria	15g
Long Gu	Dragon Bone	15g

■ Preparation

Use as prepared form or decoction with properly reduced dosage. Xi Jiao may be substituted by Shui Niu Jiao(Horn of Water Buffalo) with a 60-150g dosage.

■ Pertaining Category

Spirit Calming with Heavy Sedative Herbs

■ Functions

Nourishes Yin and blood, sedates the heart, calms spirit.

■ Indications

Yin and blood deficiency of the liver and kidney with raised liver Yang disturbing the spirit manifested as insomnia, dream disturbed sleep, palpitation, dizziness, blurred vision, red tongue with crack, scanty or thin yellow coat, a wiry, thin, or rapid pulse.

■ Cautions and Contraindications

None noted.

■ Modern Applications

Neurasthenia, paroxysmal tachycardia, etc.

Zheng Qi Tian Xiang San-Qi Correcting Cyperus Powder
Lindera and Cyperus Combination
正气天香散

■ Ingredients

Wu Yao	Lindera	9g
Xiang Fu	Cyperus Tuber	9g
Gan Jiang	Dried Ginger	9g
Zi Su Zi	Perilla Seed	9g
Chen Pi	Tangerine Seed	6g

■ **Preparation**
Use as prepared form or decoction.

■ **Pertaining Category**
Qi Regulating(Moving)

■ **Functions**
Warms the middle burner, dispels cold. Regulates Qi, alleviates pain

■ **Indications**
Qi stagnation in the middle burner due to cold manifested as acute and sudden epigastric and abdominal pain that is decreased by warmth and increased by cold, absence of thirst, clear and copious urine, loose stools, white moist tongue coat, a deep, tight pulse.

■ **Cautions and Contraindications**
It is contraindicated in cases of heat in the middle burner or where there is bleeding.

■ **Modern Applications**
Gastritis, peptic ulcer, etc.

Zhi Bai Di Huang Wan-Anemarrhena, Phellodendron, and Rehmannia Pill
Anemarrhena, Phellodendron, and Rehmannia Formula
知 柏 地 黄 丸

■ Ingredients

Shu Di Huang	Cooked Rehmannia	24g
Shan Zhu Yu	Dogwood Fruit	12g
Shan Yao	Dioscorea	12g
Fu Ling	Hoelen/Poria	9g
Ze Xie	Alisma	9g
Mu Dan Pi	Moutan Bark	9g
Zhi Mu	Anemarrhena	6g
Huang Bai	Phellodendron Bark	6g

■ Preparation
Use as prepared form or decoction.

■ Pertaining Category
Yin Tonifying

■ Functions
Nourishes the liver and kidney Yin, reduces the deficient fire. Clears damp-heat in the lower burner.

■ Indications
Yin deficiency of the liver and kidney with deficient fire marked by lower grade fever or steaming bone fever, irritability, night sweats, a feverish sensation in the palms and soles, soreness and weakness of lower back, nocturnal emission, toothache with loose teeth, or scanty and difficult urination, red tongue with scanty coat, or thin yellow coat in the back of the tongue, a thin, rapid, and empty pulse.

■ Cautions and Contraindications
Use with extreme caution for patients with indigestion and diarrhea due to deficiency of the spleen and stomach.

■ Modern Applications
Diabetes, hypertension, arteriosclerosis, hyperthyroidism, neurasthenia, chronic nephritis, chronic pyelonephritis, chronic UTI, pulmonary tuberculosis, optic neuritis or atrophy, infantile dysplasia amenorrhea, menopausal syndrome, chronic toothache, etc.

425

Zhi Bao Dan-Greatest Treasure Elixir
Rhinoceros and Amber Formula
至宝丹

■ **Ingredients**

Xi Jiao	*Rhinoceros Horn*	20-30g
She Xiang	*Musk*	0.3g
Bing Pian	*Borneol*	0.3g
An Xi Xiang	*Benzoin*	30-45g
Niu Huang	*Ox Gallstone*	12-15g
Dai Mao	*Hawksbill Shell*	20-30g
Zhu Sha	*Cinnabar*	20-30g
Hu Po	*Amber*	20-30g
Xiong Huang	*Realgar*	20-30g

■ **Preparation**
Use as prepared form.

■ **Pertaining Category**
Aromatically Opening Orifices with Cold Nature

■ **Functions**
Transforms turbid phlegm, opens orifices, induces resuscitation.
Clears heat, relieves toxicity.

■ **Indications**
Interior phlegm-heat misting the heart manifested as fever,
restlessness, delirium, impaired spirit, or coma, abundant
expectoration with harsh breathing, or infantile convulsion, red
tongue with yellow thick greasy coat, a slippery, rapid pulse.

■ Cautions and Contraindications
Do not use overdose and for long term. Do not use during pregnancy.

■ Modern Applications
Encephalitis B, cerebral vascular accident, hepatic coma, infantile convulsion, severe pneumonia, epilepsy, sunstroke in the summer, coma due to hysteria, etc.

Zhi Dai Fang(Tang)-Stop Discharge Formula(Decoction)
Stop Leukorrhea Decoction
止带方 (汤)

■ Ingredients

Zhu Ling	Polyporus	9g
Fu Ling	Hoelen/Poria	9g
Che Qian Zi	Plantago Seed	12g
Ze Xie	Alisma	9g
Yin Chen Hao	Oriental Wormwood	9g
Chi Shao Yao	Red Peony	9g
Mu Dan Pi	Moutan Bark	9g
Huang Bai	Phellodendron Bark	9g
Zhi Zi	Gardenia Fruit	9g
Niu Xi	Achyranthes	6g

■ Preparation
Use as decoction or prepared form. Che Qian Zi should be wrapped in gauze when making decoction.

■ Pertaining Category
Additional Formulas for Ob-Gyn Disorders

■ Functions
Clears heat, drains dampness, stops vaginal discharge.

Indications

Leukorrhea due to downward flowing damp-heat manifested as excessive thick, sticky, yellow or yellowish white colored vaginal discharge with foul smelling, or tinged with blood, itching in the genital area, a fullness sensation in the chest, a slimy feeling in the mouth, or lower abdominal pain, dark and scanty urine, red tongue with yellow greasy coat, a soft, rapid pulse.

Cautions and Contraindications

Use with extreme caution for patients with spleen and stomach deficiency.

Modern Applications

Leukorrhea, inflammation of the genital system, vaginitis, cervicitis etc.

Zhi Gan Cao Tang (Fu Mai Tang)-Honey Baked Licorice Decoction (Restore the Pulse Decoction)

Baked Licorice Combination
炙甘草汤 (复脉汤)

Ingredients

Zhi Gan Cao	Baked Licorice	12g
Ren Shen	Ginseng	6g
Gui Zhi	Cinnamon Twig	9g
Sheng Di Huang	Dried Rehmannia	30g
E Jiao	Equus/Gelatin	6g
Mai Men Dong	Ophiopogon	10g
Huo Ma Ren	Hemp Seed	10g
Sheng Jiang	Fresh Ginger	9g
Da Zao	Jujube	5-10pcs

Preparation

Use as decoction or prepared form. E Jiao should be dissolved separately in boiling water and added into the strained decoction.

Pertaining Category

Qi and Blood Tonifying

Functions

Tonifies Qi, nourishes Yin and blood, restores pulse.

Indications

Deficiency of Qi, blood, and Yin manifested as palpitation, shortness of breath, fatigue, insomnia, irritability, anxiety, spontaneous or night sweats, dry mouth and throat, dry stools, or dry cough with scanty, blood tinged sputum, lusterless complexion light red and dry tongue with thin coat, a intermittent, slow and uneven, or feeble and rapid pulse.

Cautions and Contraindications

It is contraindicated in cases of diarrhea due to deficiency of the spleen and stomach.

Modern Applications

Arrhythmia, extrasystole, viral myocarditis, cardiovascular neurosis rheumatic heart disease, hyperthyroidism, neurasthenia, chronic consumptive diseases, etc.

Zhi Shi Dao Zhi Wan-Guide Out Stagnation with Immature Bitter Orange Pill
Chih-shih and Rhubarb Formula
枳实导滞丸

■ Ingredients

Da Huang	*Rhubarb*	30g
Zhi Shi	*Immature Citrus*	15g
Shen Qu	*Medicated Leaven*	15g
Fu Ling	*Hoelen/Poria*	9g
Huang Qin	*Scute*	9g
Huang Lian	*Coptis*	9g
Bai Zhu	*White Atractylodes*	9g
Ze Xie	*Alisma*	6g

■ Preparation
Use as prepared form or decoction with properly adjusted dosage.

■ Pertaining Category
Food Stagnation Relieving

■ Functions
Promotes digestion, removes food stagnation. Clears heat, eliminates dampness.

■ Indications
Food stagnation with damp-heat retention manifested as distention and pain in the epigastrium and abdomen, belching or vomiting, loss of appetite, dysentery with tenesmus, odorous diarrhea with mucus, or constipation, dark and scanty urine, red tongue with yellow greasy coat, a deep, slippery, rapid, and forceful pulse.

■ Cautions and Contraindications
It is contraindicated during pregnancy and in cases of food stagnation with spleen deficiency.

■ Modern Applications
Acute gastroenteritis, acute dysentery, indigestion, acute or chronic cholecystitis, acute pancreatitis, hepatitis, etc.

Zhi Shi Xiao Pi Wan-Immature Bitter Orange Pill to Relieve Focal Distention

Relieve Focal Distention Pill with Chih-shih

枳 实 消 痞 丸

■ Ingredients

Gan Jiang	Dried Ginger	3g
Mai Ya	Barley Sprout	6g
Fu Ling	Hoelen/Poria	6g
Bai Zhu	White Atractylodes	6g
Ban Xia	Pinellia Tuber	9g
Ren Shen	Ginseng	9g
Hou Po	Magnolia Bark	12g
Zhi Shi	Immature Citrus	12g
Huang Lian	Coptis	6g
Zhi Gan Cao	Baked Licorice	6g

■ Preparation
Use as decoction or prepared form.

■ Pertaining Category
Food Stagnation Relieving

■ Functions
Relieves stuffiness and fullness. Tonifies the spleen Qi, harmonizes the stomach.

■ Indications
Spleen Qi deficiency with Qi/food stagnation and complicated cold/heat signs manifested as epigastric stuffiness, poor appetite, lassitude, abdominal distention, hesitant bowel movement, or alternating constipation and diarrhea, pale tongue with thin yellow greasy coat, a slippery pulse.

- **Cautions and Contraindications**

It is contraindicated in cases of stuffiness and focal distention of excess type.

- **Modern Applications**

Chronic gastroenteritis, chronic dysentery, intestinal dysfunction, indigestion, etc.

Zhi Shi Xie Bai Gui Zhi Tang-Immature Bitter Orange, Macrostem Onion, and Cinnamon Twig Decoction
枳实薤白桂枝汤

- **Ingredients**

Zhi Shi	*Immature Citurs*	12g
Xie Bai	*Macrostem Onion*	9g
Hou Po	*Magnolia Bark*	12g
Gui Zhi	*Cinnamon Twig*	6g
Gua Lou	*Trichosanthes Fruit*	12g

- **Preparation**

Use as decoction or prepared form.

- **Pertaining Category**

Qi Regulating(Moving)

- **Functions**

Circulates Yang Qi in the chest, expands the chest. Resolves phlegm, disperses accumulation. Descends the adverse flow of Qi.

- **Indications**

Phlegm accumulating in the chest with Qi stagnation manifested as chest fullness and pain, or even referring to the shoulder and back, cough with sputum, shortness of breath, difficulty in breathing, white greasy tongue coat, a deep, wiry, and tight pulse.

432

■ **Cautions and Contraindications**
It is contraindicated in cases of Yin deficiency with internal heat.

■ **Modern Applications**
Angina pectoris of coronary heart disease, intercostal neuralgia, chronic bronchitis, etc.

Zhi Sou San-Relieving Cough Powder
Platycodon and Schizonepeta Formula
止 嗽 散

■ **Ingredients**

Jie Geng	Platycodon	1000g
Jing Jie	Schizonepeta	1000g
Zi Wan	Purple Aster Root	1000g
Bai Bu	Stemona Root	1000g
Bai Qian	Cynanchum Root	1000g
Chen Pi	Tangerine Peel	500g
Gan Cao	Licorice	375g

■ **Preparation**
Use as prepared form or decoction with properly reduced dosage.

■ **Pertaining Category**
Treating Wind-phlegm

■ **Functions**
Expels wind, releases the exterior. Opens the lungs, resolves phlegm, stops coughing.

■ **Indications**
External wind invading the lungs with internal phlegm manifested as cough with excessive white sputum, itching throat, or slight chill and fever, thin white tongue coat, a superficial, slippery pulse.

■ **Cautions and Contraindications**
It is contraindicated in cases of cough due to lung heat, phlegm-fire, and Yin deficiency.

■ **Modern Applications**
Common cold, influenza, bronchitis, whooping cough, early stage of viral pneumonia, etc.

Zhi Zhu Wan-Immature Bitter Orange and Atractylodes Pill
Immature Bitter Orange and Atractylodes Combination
枳 术 丸

■ **Ingredients**

Zhi Shi	*Immature Citrus*	30g
Bai Zhu	*White Atractylodes*	60g

■ **Preparation**
Use as prepared form or decoction with properly reduced dosage.

■ **Pertaining Category**
Food Stagnation Relieving

■ **Functions**
Tonifies the spleen, relieves abdominal distention.

■ **Indications**
Mild spleen Qi deficiency with Qi and food stagnation manifested as epigastric and abdominal distention, poor appetite, loose stools, pale tongue with white or yellowish greasy coat, a slippery pulse.

■ **Cautions and Contraindications**
None noted.

■ **Modern Applications**
Indigestion, gastroenteritis, chronic gastritis, gastric ptosis, etc.

434

Zhi Zi Dou Chi Tang-Gardenia and Prepared Soybean Decoction

Gardenia and Prepared Soybean Combination
栀子豆豉汤

■ **Ingredients**

Zhi Zi	Gardenia	9g
Dan Dou Chi	Prepared Soybean	9g

■ **Preparation**
Use as decoction or prepared form.

■ **Pertaining Category**
Qi Level Heat Clearing

■ **Functions**
Clears heat, relieves irritability.

■ **Indications**
Heat in the Qi level manifested as fever, restlessness, irritability, insomnia, a stifling sensation in the chest, red tip tongue with yellow coat, a rapid, full pulse.

■ **Cautions and Contraindications**
This formula may cause vomiting.

■ **Modern Applications**
Unexplained fever, upper respiratory tract infection, pneumonia, gastritis, neurosis, neurasthenia, etc.

Zhong Man Fen Xiao Wan-Middle Burner Fullness Separating and Reducing Pill
中满分消丸

■ Ingredients

Hou Po	Magnolia Bark	15g
Zhi Shi	Immature Citrus	15g
Huang Lian	Coptis	6g
Huang Qin	Scute	9g
Zhi Mu	Anemarrhena	12g
Ban Xia	Pinellia Tuber	15g
Chen Pi	Tangerine Peel	9g
Fu Ling	Hoelen/Poria	6g
Zhu Ling	Polyporus	3g
Ze Xie	Alisma	9g
Sha Ren	Amomum Fruit	6g
Gan Jiang	Dried Ginger	6g
Jiang Huang	Turmeric Rhizome	3g
Ren Shen	Ginseng	3g
Bai Zhu	White Atractylodes	3g
Zhi Gan Cao	Baked Licorice	3g

■ Preparation
Use as prepared form or decoction with properly adjusted dosage.

■ Pertaining Category
Additional Formulas for Internal Medicine

■ Functions
Clears heat, drains dampness. Regulates Qi. Strengthens the spleen

■ Indications
Damp-heat obstructing in the middle burner with underlying spleen Qi deficiency manifested as fullness, hardness, and pain in the epigastrium and abdomen, irritability, fever, a bitter taste in the mouth, thirst, dark and difficult urine, foul-smelling diarrhea, or jaundice, red sides and tip tongue with yellow greasy coat, a wiry, rapid pulse.

■ **Cautions and Contraindications**

It should be only used with modification for condition due to cold.

■ **Modern Applications**

Ascites from liver cirrhosis, etc.

Zhou Che Wan-Vessel and Vehicle Pill
Kansui and Pharbitis Formula
舟 车 丸

■ **Ingredients**

Qian Niu Zi	*Pharbitis Seed*	120g
Gan Sui	*Kansui*	30g
Yuan Hua	*Daphne Flower*	30g
Da Ji	*Euphorbia*	30g
Da Huang	*Rhubarb*	60g
Qing Pi	*Green Citrus Peel*	15g
Chen Pi	*Tangerine Peel*	15g
Mu Xiang	*Saussurea*	15g
Bing Lang	*Areca Seed*	15g
Qing Fen	*Calomelas*	3g

■ **Preparation**

Use as powder or pill form. Grind all ingredients into powder and make pills with water, take 3-6g with warm water on an empty stomach in the morning for one time.

■ **Pertaining Category**

Purging Downward with Harsh Cathartics

■ **Functions**

Promotes the movement of Qi, harshly eliminates accumulated water and heat.

437

■ Indications

Severe interior water and heat accumulation obstructing Qi manifested as severe edema, water retention, thirst, a hard abdomen, difficult and coarse breathing, constipation, scanty urine, red tongue with greasy coat, a deep, rapid, and forceful pulse.

■ Cautions and Contraindications

It is contraindicated for pregnant women and patients with weak constitution.

■ Modern Applications

Edema, ascites from liver cirrhosis, schistosomiasis, etc.
This formula is highly toxic, only a strong patient may take a reduced dosage for 1-2 days more if necessary.

Zhu Ling Tang-Polyporus Decoction
Polyporus Combination
猪 苓 汤

■ Ingredients

Zhu Ling	Polyporus	9g
Fu Ling	Hoelen/Poria	9g
Ze Xie	Alisma Tuber	9g
E Jiao	Equus/Gelatin	9g
Hua Shi	Talcum	9g

■ Preparation

Use as decoction or prepared form. E Jiao should be dissolved separately in boiling water and added into the strained decoction.

■ Pertaining Category

Downward Dampness Draining

■ Functions

Induces diuresis. Clears heat. Nourishes Yin.

■ **Indications**

Water accumulating in the lower burner with heat and injured Yin manifested as fever, thirst with a desire to drink water, painful and difficult urination, urinary bleeding, distending pain in the lower abdomen, or irritability, insomnia, or nausea, diarrhea, and cough, red tongue with thin yellow greasy coat, a rapid pulse.

■ **Cautions and Contraindications**

Use very cautiously for patients with high fever, excessive sweating, and severe damage of Yin.

■ **Modern Applications**

Mild case of UTI, lithangiuria, nephritis, gastroenteritis, etc.

Zhu Sha An Shen Wan-Cinnabar Sedative Pill

Cinnabar Formula

朱 砂 安 神 丸

■ **Ingredients**

Zhu Sha	Cinnabar	15g
Huang Lian	Coptis	18g
Sheng Di Huang	Dried Rehmannia	8g
Dang Gui	Chinese Angelica	8g
Zhi Gan Cao	Baked Licorice	16g

■ **Preparation**

Use as prepared form.

■ **Pertaining Category**

Spirit Calming with Heavy Sedative Herbs

■ **Functions**

Calms spirit, relieves palpitation. Clears heat. Nourishes blood and Yin.

■ **Indications**

Heart fire flaming up with insufficient heart blood and Yin manifested as palpitation, restlessness, insomnia, dream disturbed sleep, an irritable heat sensation in the chest, nausea, forgetfulness, red tongue, a thin, rapid pulse.

■ **Cautions and Contraindications**

Do not use overdose and for long term to prevent mercurialism from Zhu Sha (Cinnabar). Do not use during pregnancy.

■ **Modern Applications**

Neurosis, neurasthenia, psychosis, mental depression, etc.

Zhu Ye Liu Bang Tang-Bamboo Leaf, Tamarix, and Burdock Seed decoction
竹叶柳蒡汤

■ **Ingredients**

Sheng Liu	Tamarix Chinensis	6g
Jing Jie Sui	Schizonepeta Spike	4.5g
Ge Gen	Pueraria	4.5g
Chan Tui	Cicada Skin	3g
Bo He	Peppermint	3g
Niu Bang Zi	Burdock Seed	4.5g
Zhi Mu	Anemarrhena	3g
Xuan Shen	Scrophularia Root	6g
Mai Men Dong	Ophiopogon	9g
Dan Zhu Ye	Bland Bamboo Leaf	1.5g
Gan Cao	Licorice	3g

■ **Preparation**

Use as decoction or prepared form. Bo He should be added 5 minutes near the end of cooking.

■ **Pertaining Category**
Pungent Cool Exterior Relieving

■ **Functions**
Disperses wind-heat, releases the exterior, promotes eruption of the measles. Clears heat from lungs and stomach. Nourishes Yin.

■ **Indications**
Early stage of the measles with exterior pathogen and interior heat manifested as rashes that do not erupt evenly, fever, lack of sweating, cough, difficulty in breathing, a stifling sensation in the chest, restlessness, sore and swollen throat, red and dry tongue, a superficial, rapid pulse.

■ **Cautions and Contraindications**
The king herb (Sheng Liu-Tamarix) has strong effect of expelling pathogen, it should not be used overdose. It should be discontinued once the rashes are erupted.

■ **Modern Applications**
Influenza, measles, measles accompanied by pneumonia, scarlet fever, etc.
For severe internal heat, Shi Gao (Gypsum)15g, Jing Mi (Oryza)15g should be added,

Zhu Ye Shi Gao Tang-Bamboo Leaf and Gypsum Decoction
Bamboo Leaf and Gypsum Combination
竹叶石膏汤

■ **Ingredients**

Dan Zhu Ye	Bland Bamboo Leaf	15g
Shi Gao	Gypsum	30g
Ban Xia	Pinellia Tuber	9g
Mai Men Dong	Ophiopogon	15g
Ren Shen	Ginseng	5g
Zhi Gan Cao	Baked Licorice	3g
Geng Mi	Oryza	15g

■ **Preparation**
Use as decoction or prepared form.

■ **Pertaining Category**
Qi Level Heat Clearing

■ **Functions**
Clears heat, promotes the generation of body fluid. Tonifies Qi, harmonizes the stomach.

■ **Indications**
Later stage of febrile disease with residual heat in Qi level and impairment of Qi and body fluids or summer heat damaging Qi and Yin manifested as mild fever, profuse sweating, shortness of breath irritability, nausea or vomiting, dry mouth with a desire to drink, or insomnia, red tongue with scanty coat, a rapid, thin, and weak pulse

■ **Cautions and Contraindications**
It is contraindicated in cases of existing excess heat without damaging Qi and Yin.

■ **Modern Applications**
Influenza, epidemic encephalitis B, epidemic cerebrospinal meningitis, pneumonia, septicemia, summer heat stroke, gingivitis, diabetes, etc.

Zi Xue Dan-Purple Snow Elixir
Rhinoceros and Antelope Horn Formula
紫血丹

- **Ingredients**

Xi Jiao	*Rhinoceros Horn*	150g
Ling Yang Jiao	*Antelope horn*	150g
She Xiang	*Musk*	1.5g
Shi Gao	*Gypsum*	1500g
Han Shui Shi	*Calcite*	1500g
Hua Shi	*Talcum*	1500g
Ci Shi	*Magnetite*	1500g
Qing Mu Xiang	*Aristolochia*	150g
Chen Xiang	*Aquilaria*	150g
Xuan Shen	*Scrophularia*	500g
Sheng Ma	*Cimicifuga*	500g
Ding Xiang	*Cloves*	30g
Mang Xiao	*Mirabilitum*	5000g
Xiao Shi	*Saltprter*	96g
Zhu Sha	*Cinnabar*	90g
Huang Jin	*Gold*	3000g
Zhi Gan Cao	*Baked Licorice*	240g

- **Preparation**

Use as prepared form only. In modern use, gold should be omitted.

- **Pertaining Category**

Aromatically Opening Orifices with Cold Nature

- **Functions**

Clears heat, relieves toxicity. Opens orifices, stops convulsion. Calms spirit.

Indications

Epidemic febrile disease with toxic-heat penetrating the pericardium and stirring-up of the liver wind manifested as high fever, restlessness, delirium, impaired spirit, convulsion, thirst with dry and parched lips, dark and scanty urine, constipation, or infantile convulsion, red tongue with yellow coat, a wiry, rapid, and forceful pulse.

Cautions and Contraindications

It is contraindicated in cases of coma due to phlegm-cold. Do not use overdose and for long term. Do not use during pregnancy.

Modern Applications

Encephalitis B, epidemic cerebrospinal meningitis, scarlet fever, severe pneumonia, measles, epilepsy, acute tonsillitis, etc.

Zuo Gui Wan-Left Restoring Pill
Cyathula and Rehmannia Formula
左 归 丸

Ingredients

Shu Di Huang	Cooked Rehmannia	240g
Shan Zhu Yu	Dogwood Fruit	120g
Shan Yao	Dioscorea	120g
Gou Qi Zi	Lycium Fruit	120g
Tu Si Zi	Dodder Seed	120g
Chuan Niu Xi	Cyathula	90g
Lu Jiao Jiao	Colloid of Antler	120g
Gui Ban Jiao	Colloid of Turtle Shell	120g

Preparation

Use as prepared form.

■ Pertaining Category
Yin Tonifying

■ Functions
Nourishes the kidney Yin and essences.

■ Indications
Deficiency of the kidney Yin and essence manifested as dizziness, blurred vision, soreness and weakness of lower back, nocturnal emission, spermatorrhea, night sweats, dry mouth and throat, thirst with a desire to drink water, loss of hair and teeth, infertility, or amenorrhea, red tongue with scanty coat, a thin, rapid pulse.

■ Cautions and Contraindications
Use with extreme caution for patients with indigestion and diarrhea due to deficiency of the spleen and stomach.

■ Modern Applications
Chronic consumptive diseases, diabetes, lumbago, tuberculosis, infertility, amenorrhea, spermatorrhea, etc.

Zuo Gui Yin-Left Restoring Beverage
Replenishing the Yin Formula
左归饮

■ Ingredients

Shu Di Huang	Cooked Rehmannia	9g
Shan Zhu Yu	Dogwood Fruit	5g
Shan Yao	Dioscorea	6g
Gou Qi Zi	Lycium Fruit	6g
Fu Ling	Hoelen/Poria	4g
Zhi Gan Cao	Baked Licorice	3g

■ Preparation
Use as decoction or prepared form.

■ Pertaining Category

Yin Tonifying

■ Functions

Nourishes the kidney and liver Yin.

■ Indications

Deficiency of the liver and kidney Yin manifested as soreness and weakness of lower back, nocturnal emission or spermatorrhea, night sweats, dry mouth and throat, thirst with a desire to drink water, dizziness, blurred vision, tinnitus, red tongue with scanty coat, a thin, rapid pulse.

■ Cautions and Contraindications

Use with caution for patients with digestive disorders.

■ Modern Applications

Lumbago, diabetes, tuberculosis, chronic UTI, glaucoma, cataract, etc.

This is a milder formula to tonify kidney Yin comparing to Liu Wei Di Huang Wan and Zuo Gui Wan.

Zuo Jin Wan-Left Metal Pill
Coptis and Evodia Pill
左金丸

■ Ingredients

| Huang Lian | *Coptis* | 180g |
| Wu Zhu Yu | *Evodia* | 15-30g |

■ Preparation

Use as prepared form or decoction with properly reduced dosage.

■ Pertaining Category

Clearing Heat from Zang-fu Organs

■ **Functions**

Clears liver fire. Descends the rebellious Qi downward, stops vomiting.

■ **Indications**

Liver fire affecting stomach manifested as hypochondriac distending pain, epigastric distention, belching, sour regurgitation, nausea, vomiting, a bitter taste in the mouth, red tongue with yellow coat, a wiry, rapid pulse.

■ **Cautions and Contraindications**

It is contraindicated in cases of acid regurgitation due to deficient cold in the middle burner.

■ **Modern Applications**

Peptic ulcer, esophageal reflux, gastritis, esophagitis, hiatal hernia, hiccups, acute dysentery, etc.

Clinical Application of
Chinese Herbal Formulas
by Differentiation According to Zang-fu Organs

Heart Syndrome	Deficiency of the heart Qi	**Yang Xin Tang**-Nourish the Heart Decoction
		Sheng Mai San-Activate the Pulse Powder
		Ding Zhi Wan-Stabilize the Emotions Pill
	Deficiency of the heart Yang	**Ren Shen Yang Rong Tang**-Ginseng Nourish Nutritive Qi Decoction
		Shi Quan Da Bu Tang-Great Tonifying Decoction with Ten Ingredients
		Zhen Wu Tang-True Warrior Decoction
	Collapse of the heart Yang	**Shen Fu Tang**-Ginseng and Aconite Decoction
		Si Ni Jia Ren Shen Tang-Four Frigid Limbs Decoction with Ginseng
	Deficiency of the heart Yin	**Tian Wang Bu Xin Dan**-Heavenly Emperor Heart Tonifying Elixir
		Bai Zi Yang Xin Wan-Biota Seed Nourishing the Heart Pill
		Zhi Gan Cao Tang-Honey Baked Licorice Decoction
	Deficiency of the heart blood	**Si Wu Tang**-Four Substances Decoction
		Gui Pi Tang-Restore the Spleen Decoction
		Zhi Gan Cao Tang-Honey Baked Licorice Decoction

Heart Syndrome (cont.)	Stagnation of the heart blood	**Gua Lou Xie Bai Ban Xia Tang-**Trichosanthes, Macrostem Onion, and Pinellia Decoction **Xue Fu Zhu Yu Tang-**Remove Stasis from the Mansion of Blood Decoction **Dan Shen Yin-**Salvia Root Beverage
	Hyperactivity of the heart fire	**Dao Chi San-**Guide Out the Red Powder **Xie Xin Tang-**Drain the Heart and Stomach Decoction **Zhu Sha An Shen Wan-**Cinnabar Sedative Pill
	Derange-ment of the mind-phlegm misting the heart	**Dao Tan Tang-**Guide Out Phlegm Decoction **Di Tan Tang-**Phlegm Flushing Decoction **Su He Xiang Wan-**Styrax Pill
	Derange-ment of the mind-phlegm fire disturbing the heart	**Gun Tan Wan-**Rolling Out Phlegm Pill **Sheng Tie Luo Yin-**Iron Filings Beverage **Wen Dan Tang-**Warm the Gallbladder Decoction
	Retention of harmful phlegm-fluid attacking the heart	**Ling Gui Zhu Gan Tang-**Poria, Cinnamon, Atractylodes, and Licorice Decoction **Zhen Wu Tang-**True Warrior Decoction
Small Intestine Syndrome	Excessive heat in the small intestine	**Dao Chi San-**Guide Out the Red Powder

Small Intestine Syndrome (cont.)	Deficient cold in the small intestine	**Li Zhong Wan**-Regulate the Middle Burner Pill
	Pain due to disturbance of the small intestine Qi	**Nuan Gan Jian**-Warm the Liver Brew **Ju He Wan**-Tangerine Seed Pill
Lung Syndrome	Invasion of the lungs by wind-cold	**Ma Huang Tang**-Ephedra Decoction **Gui Zhi Tang**-Cinnamon Twig Decoction **Jia Wei Xiang Su San**-Augmented Cyperus and Perilla Leaf Powder **Jing Fang Bai Du San**-Schizonepeta and Siler Powder to Overcome Toxicity
	Invasion of the lungs by wind-heat	**Sang Ju Yin**-Mulberry Leaf and Chrysanthemum Beverage **Yin Qiao San**-Lonicera Flower and Forsythia Powder **Chai Ge Jie Ji Tang**-Bupleurum and Pueraria Release Muscle Layer Decoction
	External dryness affecting the lungs	**Xing Su San**-Apricot Seed and Perilla Powder **Sang Xing Tang**-Morus and Apricot Seed decoction **Qing Zao Jiu Fei Tang**-Clear Dryness and Rescue the Lung Decoction
	Excessive heat in the lungs	**Ma Huang Xing Ren Gan Cao Shi Gao Tang**-Ephedra, Apricot Seed, Licorice, and Gypsum Decoction **Wei Jing Tang**-Reed Decoction

Lung Syndrome (cont.)	Retention of phlegm-damp in the lungs	**Er Chen Tang**-Two Matured Ingredients Decoction
		Xiao Qing Long Tang-Minor Bluegreen Dragon Decoction
		San Zi Yang Qin Tang-Three Seeds Nourishing the Parents Decoction
		She Gan Ma Huang Tang-Belamcanda and Ephedra Decoction
	Retention of phlegm-heat in the lungs	**Qing Qi Hua Tan Wan**-Clear Qi and Resolve Phlegm Decoction
		Ding Chuan Tang-Arrest Wheezing Decoction
		Xiao Xian Xiong Tang-Minor Sinking into Chest Decoction
		Wei Jing Tang-Reed Decoction
	Deficiency of the lung Qi	**Bu Fei Tang**-Tonify the Lungs Decoction
		Liu Jun Zi Tang-Six Gentleman Decoction
		Ren Shen Ge Jie San-Ginseng and Gecko Powder
		Yu Ping Feng San-Jade Screen Powder
	Deficiency of the lung Yin	**Sha Shen Mai Men Dong Tang**-Glehnia and Ophiopogon Decoction
		Bai He Gu Jin Tang-Lily Bulb Decoction to Consolidate the Metal
		Bu Fei E Jiao Tang-Tonify the Lungs Decoction with Donkey-hide Gelatin

Large Intestine Syndrome	Damp-heat in the large intestine	**Ge Gen Huang Qin Huang Lian Tang**-Pueraria, Scute, and Coptis Decoction
		Shao Yao Tang-Peony Decoction
		Bai Tou Weng Tang-Pulsatilla Decoction
	Consumption of the fluids in the large intestine	**Ma Zi Ren Wan**-Hemp Seed Pill
		Run Chang Wan-Moisten the Intestines Pill
		Zeng Ye Cheng Qi Tang-Increase the Fluids and Purge Down Digestive Qi Decoction
Spleen Syndrome	Deficiency of the spleen Qi	**Si Jun Zi Tang**-Four Gentleman Decoction
		Liu Jun Zi Tang-Six Gentleman Decoction
		Xiang Sha Liu Jun Zi Tang-Saussurea, Amomum, and Six Gentleman Decoction
		Shen Ling Bai Zhu San-Ginseng, Hoelen, and White Atractylodes Powder
		Xiao Jian Zhong Tang-Minor Strengthen the Middle Burner Decoction
		Huang Qi Jian Zhong Tang-Astragalus Strengthen the Middle Burner Decoction

Spleen Syndrome (cont.)	Deficiency of the spleen Yang	**Li Zhong Wan**-Regulate the Middle Burner Pill
		Fu Zi Li Zhong Wan(Tang) -Regulate the Middle Burner Pill(Decoction) with Aconite
		Da Jian Zhong Tang-Major Strengthen the Middle Burner Decoction
		Shi Pi San (Yin) -Bolster the Spleen Powder (Beverage)
	Dysfunction of the spleen in controlling blood	**Gui Pi Tang**-Restore the Spleen Decoction
		Huang Tu Tang-Baked Yellow Earth Decoction
		Gu Chong Tang-Stabilize Gushing Decoction
		Gu Ben Zhi Beng Tang-Secure Root and Stop Uterine Bleeding Decoction
	Sinking of the spleen Qi	**Bu Zhong Yi Qi Tang**-Reinforce the Middle Burner and Tonify Qi Decoction
		Sheng Xian Tang-Raise the Sinking Decoction
		Ju Yuan Jian-Lift the Source Decoction
	Invasion of the spleen by damp-cold	**Wei Ling Tang**-Stomach Calming and Hoelen Five Decoction
		Ping Wei San-Calm the Stomach Powder
		Hou Po Wen Zhong Tang-Magnolia Bark Decoction to Warm the Middle Burner

Spleen Syndrome (cont.)	Damp-heat in the middle burner	**Gan Lu Xiao Du Dan**-Sweet Dew Toxin-Eliminating Elixir
		Yin Chen Hao Tang-Capillaris Decoction
Stomach Syndrome	Cold in the stomach	**Da Jian Zhong Tang**-Major Strengthen the Middle Burner Decoction
		Li Zhong Wan-Regulate the Middle Burner Pill
		Liang Fu Wan-Galanga and Cyperus Pill
		Ding Xiang Shi Di Tang-Cloves and Kaki Decoction
	Hyperactivity of fire in the stomach	**Qing Wei San**-Clear the Stomach Powder
		Xie Xin Tang-Drain the Heart and Stomach Decoction
		Tiao Wei Cheng Qi Tang-Regulate Stomach Decoction for Purging Down Digestive Qi
	Retention of food in the stomach	**Bao He Wan**-Preserving Harmony Pill
		Zhi Shi Dao Zhi Wan-Guide Out Stagnation with Immature Bitter Orange Pill
	Insufficiency of the stomach Yin	**Yu Nu Jian**-Jade Woman Brew
		Yi Wei Tang-Benefit the Stomach Decoction
		Sha Shen Mai Men Dong Tang-Glehnia and Ophiopogon Decoction
		Mai Men Dong Tang-Ophiopogon Decoction

Liver Syndrome	Stagnation of the liver Qi	**Si Ni San**-Powder for Treating Cold Limbs
		Chai Hu Shu Gan San-Bupleurum Powder to Disperse Liver Qi
		Jin Ling Zi San-Melia Toosandan Powder
		Xiao Yao San-Wandering Powder
		Ban Xia Hou Po Tang-Pinellia and Magnolia Bark Decoction
	Flare-up of the liver fire	**Jia Wei Xiao Yao San**-Augmented Wandering Powder
		Long Dan Xie Gan Tang-Gentiana Drain the Liver Decoction
		Dang Gui Long Hui Wan-Tang-kuei, Gentiana, and Aloe Pill
	Raising of the liver Yang	**Tian Ma Gou Teng Yin**-Gastrodia and Uncaria Beverage
		Qi Ju Di Huang Wan-Lycium, Chrysanthemum, and Rehmannia Pill
	Stirring of the liver wind in the interior	**Zhen Gan Xi Feng Tang**-Sedate the Liver and Extinguish Wind Decoction
		Ling Jiao Gou Teng Tang-Antelope Horn and Uncaria Decoction
		Da Ding Feng Zhu-Major Arrest Wind Pearl

Liver Syndrome (cont.)	Damp-heat in the liver and gall-bladder	**Long Dan Xie Gan Tang**-Gentiana Drain the Liver Decoction **Yin Chen Hao Tang**-Capillaris Decoction **Hao Qin Qing Dan Tang**-Sweet Wormwood and Scute Decoction to Clear the Gallbladder
	Insufficiency of the liver blood	**Si Wu Tang**-Four Substances Decoction **Bu Gan Tang**-Tonify the Liver Decoction **Qi Bao Mei Ran Dan**-Seven Treasure Elixir for Beautiful Whiskers
	Deficiency of the liver Yin	**Yi Guan Jian**-Linking Brew **Qi Ju Di Huang Wan**-Lycium, Chrysanthemum, and Rehmannia Pill
	Retention of cold in the liver channel	**Nuan Gan Jian**-Warm the Liver Brew **Tian Tai Wu Yao San**-Heaven Stage Lindera Powder
Gallbladder Syndrome	Gallbladder disharmony with phlegm-heat retention	**Wen Dan Tang**-Warm the Gallbladder Decoction **Hao Qin Qing Dan Tang**-Sweet Wormwood and Scute Decoction to Clear the Gallbladder
Kidney Syndrome	Kidney Yang deficiency	**Jin Gui Shen Qi Wan**-Tonify the Kidney Qi Pill from Golden Cabinet **You Gui Wan**-Right Restoring Pill **You Gui Yin**-Right Restoring Beverage **Zhen Wu Tang**-True Warrior Decoction

Kidney Syndrome (cont.)	Kidney Yin deficiency	**Liu Wei Di Huang Wan**-Six Ingredients Pill with Rehmannia
		Zhi Bai Di Huang Wan-Anemarrhena, Phellodendron, and Rehmannia Pill
		Qi Ju Di Huang Wan-Lycium, Chrysanthemum, and Rehmannia Pill
		Ba Xian Chang Shou Wan-Eight Immortal Longevity Pill
		Zuo Gui Wan-Left Restoring Pill
		Zuo Gui Yin-Left Restoring Beverage
	Kidney failing to grasp Qi	**Ren Shen Hu Tao Tang**-Ginseng and Walnut Decoction
		Su Zi Jiang Qi Tang-Perilla Seed Descending Qi Decoction
	Insufficiency of the kidney essence	**He Che Da Zao Wan**-Major Tonifying Pill with Human Placenta
		Qi Bao Mei Ran Dan-Seven Treasure Elixir for Beautiful Whiskers
	Kidney failing to consolidate Qi and essence	**Jin Suo Gu Jing Wan**-Golden Lock Stabilizing Essence Pill
		Suo Quan Wan-Reduce Stream Pill
Urinary Bladder Syndrome	Damp-heat in the bladder	**Ba Zheng San**-Eight Straight Powder
		Shi Wei San-Pyrrosia Leaf Powder
		Er Miao San-Two Marvel Powder
		Bei Xie Fen Qing Yin II-Hypoglauca Yam Beverage to Separate Clear from Turbid

Clinical Application of Chinese Herbal Formulas
by Differentiation According to Six Stages

Taiyang Stage	Channel Syndrome	Zhong Feng Zheng (Attacked by wind with exterior deficiency)	**Gui Zhi Tang-**Cinnamon Twig Decoction
		Shang Han Zheng (Attacked by cold with exterior excess)	**Ma Huang Tang-**Ephedra Decoction
			Ge Gen Tang-Pueraria Decoction
			Da Qing Long Tang-Major Bluegreen Dragon Decoction
			Xiao Qing Long Tang-Minor Bluegreen Dragon Decoction
	Fu Syndrome	Xu Shui Zheng (Water accumulating in the bladder)	**Wu Ling San-**Five Ingredients Powder with Poria
		Xu Xue Zheng (Stagnant blood in the lower abdomen)	**Tao He Cheng Qi Tang-**Persica Seed Decoction for Purging Down Digestive Qi
Shaoyang Stage			**Xiao Chai Hu Tang-**Minor Bupleurum Decoction

Shaoyang Stage (cont.)			**Da Chai Hu Tang**-Major Bupleurum Decoction
			Chai Hu Gui Zhi Tang-Bupleurum and Cinnamon Twig Decoction
			Chai Hu Jia Long Gu Mu Li Tang-Bupleurum Plus Dragon Bone and Oyster Shell Decoction
Yangming Stage	Channel Syndrome		**Bai Hu Tang**-White Tiger Decoction
			Bai Hu Jia Ren Shen Tang-White Tiger Plus Ginseng Decoction
			Zhu Ye Shi Gao Tang-Bamboo Leaf and Gypsum Decoction

Yangming Stage (cont.)	Fu Syndrome		**Da Cheng Qi Tang-** Major Decoction for Purging Down Digestive Qi
			Xiao Cheng Qi Tang- Minor Decoction for Purging Down Digestive Qi
			Tiao Wei Cheng Qi Tang- Regulate Stomach Decoction for Purging Down Digestive Qi
			Ma Zi Ren Wan- Hemp Seed Pill
Taiyin Stage			**Li Zhong Wan-** Regulate the Middle Burner Pill

Shaoyin Stage		Xu Han Zheng (Deficient cold pattern)	**Si Ni Tang**-Four Frigid Limbs Decoction
			Si Ni Jia Ren Shen Tang-Four Frigid Limbs Decoction with Ginseng
			Tong Mai Si Ni Tang-Unblock the Channel Decoction for Four Frigid Limbs
			Zhen Wu Tang-True Warrior Decoction
		Xu Re Zheng (Deficient heat pattern)	**Huang Lian E Jiao Tang**-Coptis and Donkey-hide Gelatin Decoction
			Zhu Ling Tang-Polyporus Decoction
Jueyin Stage			**Wu Mei Wan**-Mume Pill
			Wu Zhu Yu Tang-Evodia Decoction

Clinical Application of Chinese Herbal Formulas
by Differentiation According to Four Levels

Heat in the Wei (Defensive) Level	Wind-heat	**Yin Qiao San**-Lonicera Flower and Forsythia Powder
		Sang Ju Yin-Mulberry Leaf and Chrysanthemum Beverage
	Wind-heat-dryness	**Sang Xing Tang**-Morus and Apricot Seed Decoction
Heat in the Qi Level	Heat in the Yangming channel	**Bai Hu Tang**-White Tiger Decoction
		Zhu Ye Shi Gao Tang-Bamboo Leaf and Gypsum Decoction
	Heat in the lungs	**Ma Huang Xing Ren Gan Cao Shi Gao Tang**-Ephedra, Apricot Seed, Licorice, and Gypsum Decoction
	Heat in the chest and diaphragm	**Zhi Zi Dou Chi Tang**-Gardenia and Prepared Soybean Decoction
		Liang Ge San-Cool the Diaphragm Powder
	Heat in the stomach and large intestine	**Da Cheng Qi Tang**-Major Decoction for Purging Down Digestive Qi
		Zeng Ye Cheng Qi Tang-Increase the Fluids and Purge Down Digestive Qi Decoction
	Heat in the liver and gallbladder	**Long Dan Xie Gan Tang**-Gentiana Drain the Liver Decoction
		Jin Ling Zi San-Melia Toosandan Powder
		Jia Wei Xiao Yao San-Augmented Wandering Powder

Heat in the Ying (Nutritive) Level		**Qing Ying Tang**-Clear the Nutritive Level Decoction
		An Gong Niu Huang Wan-Calm the Palace Pill with Ox Gallstone
		Zi Xue Dan-Purple Snow Elixir
		Zhi Bao Dan-Greatest Treasure Elixir
Heat in the Blood Level		**Xi Jiao Di Huang Tang**-Rhinoceros Horn and Rehmannia Decoction
		Ling Jiao Gou Teng Tang-Antelope Horn and Uncaria Decoction
		San Jia Fu Mai Tang-Three Shells Decoction to Restore the Pulse
		Da Ding Feng Zhu-Major Arrest Wind Pearl
Heat in the Qi and Blood Level		**Qing Wen Bai Du Yin**-Clear Epidemics and Antitoxin Beverage

Application of Chinese Herbal Formulas
by Differentiation According to Triple Burners

Damp-heat in the Upper Burner	**Huo Xiang Zheng Qi San**-Agastache Qi Rectifying Powder
	Huo Po Xia Ling Tang-Agastache, Magnolia Bark, Pinellia, and Poria Decoction
Damp-heat in the Middle Burner	**Gan Lu Xiao Du Dan**-Sweet Dew Toxin Eliminating Elixir
	San Ren Tang-Three Seeds Decoction
	Yin Chen Hao Tang-Capillaris Decoction
	Wen Dan Tang-Warm the Gallbladder Decoction
Damp-heat in the Lower Burner	**Fu Ling Pi Tang**-Hoelen Peel Decoction
	Ba Zheng San-Eight Straight Powder
	Ge Gen Huang Qin Huang Lian Tang-Pueraria, Scute, and Coptis Decoction
	Shao Yao Tang-Peony Decoction
	Bai Tou Weng Tang-Pulsatilla Decoction

Bibliography

Chinese Herbal Medicine-Formula & Strategies
Dan Bensky & Randall Barolet
Eastland Press, Inc., 1990, Seattle, WA

Handbook of Chinese Herbs and Formulas
Him-che Yeung
Institute of Chinese Medicine, 1985, Los Angeles, CA

Prescription of Traditional Chinese Medicine
Enqin Zhang
Publishing House of Shanghai College of Traditional Chinese
Medicine, 1988, Shanghai, China

Chinese Herbalist's Handbook
Dagmar Ehling
Inword Press, 1994, Santa Fe, NM

Chinese Herbal formula
Ji Qun Xu
Shanghai Science and Technology Press, 1985, Shanghai, China

Chinese herbs and Formulas
Meng Jun Huang
Traditional Chinese Medicine Press, 1998, Beijing, China

Brief Chinese Medicine dictionary
Editorial board
People's Health Press, 1979, Beijing, China

Chinese Acupuncture and Moxibustion
Xinnong Cheng
Foreign Languages Press, 1987, Beijing, China